AUTISM
Through
A SENSORY LENS

The fully revised second edition of this easy-to-use resource introduces the sensory differences autistic children may face, and explores how these differences can affect their ability to make sense of the world. It is invaluable in helping those adults working with autistic children to identify the possible triggers for the child's behaviour and consider it through *a sensory lens.*

Children have varying sensory needs so the book offers both a wealth of enjoyable activities for sensory exploration and play, whilst also providing suggestions for strategies and ideas that can be used at home or in school to create an autism-friendly environment.

This book:

- Highlights the possible link between behaviours that challenge and sensory difficulties for autistic children.

- Provides practical and accessible resources, helping parents, carers and practitioners to gain a greater understanding of sensory differences.

- Includes an online assessment with accompanying aids to create a visual representation of the child's sensory needs.

With both downloadable and photocopiable resources, this practical guide will be an essential tool for parents, carers and practitioners working with children with autism, enabling them to create a visual profile of areas of difficulty which can form the basis of personalised strategies and fun sensory activities to support the child.

Joy Beaney has over 30 years of teaching experience in both mainstream and special education. Joy lectures at Brighton University, delivering its Post Graduate Certificate in autism. Her consultancy work, training, conferences and publishing all contribute to supporting individuals and organisations to make the world a more autism-friendly place.

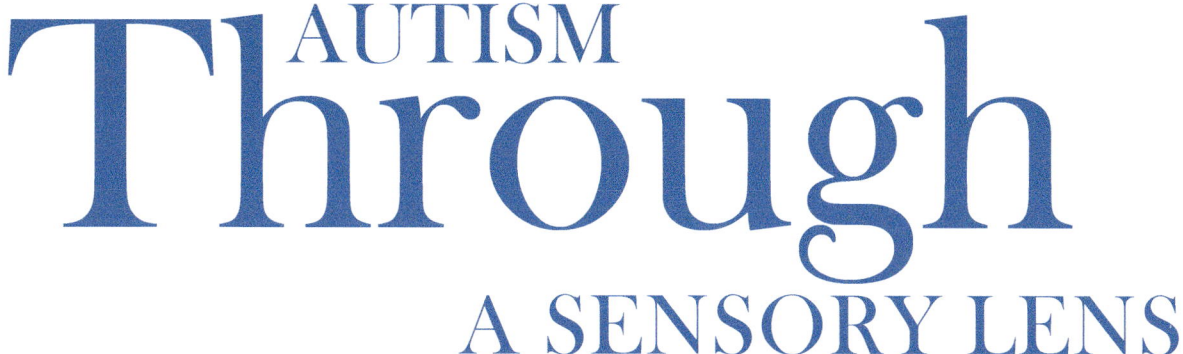

AUTISM
Through
A SENSORY LENS

Sensory Assessment and Strategies

2

JOY BEANEY

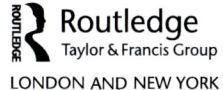

Routledge
Taylor & Francis Group

LONDON AND NEW YORK

Second edition published 2021
by Routledge
2 Park Square, Milton Park, Abingdon, Oxon, OX14 4RN

and by Routledge
52 Vanderbilt Avenue, New York, NY 10017

Routledge is an imprint of the Taylor & Francis Group, an informa business

© 2021 Joy Beaney

First edition published by Speechmark 2013

British Library Cataloguing-in-Publication Data
A catalogue record for this book is available from the British Library

Library of Congress Cataloging-in-Publication Data
A catalog record for this book has been requested

ISBN: 978-0-367-50266-9 (hbk)
ISBN: 978-0-367-36962-0 (pbk)
ISBN: 978-0-429-35208-9 (ebk)

Typeset in Frutiger
by Apex CoVantage, LLC

Visit the companion website: www.routledge.com/cw/speechmark

Contents

Acknowledgements

My thanks to colleagues I have worked with over the years for their support and encouragement. I would particularly like to thank Kay Al-Ghani for her inspiration and encouragement and her son Haitham for the delightful illustrations he has designed and drawn for this book.

I would also like to thank the parents for sharing insights into their children which proved invaluable in the development of this sensory resource.

Finally, and most importantly, I would like to thank the amazing children who I have worked with and who have inspired me to develop this resource.

Introduction: *autism through a sensory lens*

We are all unique and the way in which autism affects the individual is variable.

The aims of this book are to help you gain a greater understanding of the child's sensory differences and that by seeing autism through a sensory lens, you can better appreciate how the child experiences the world. Each child will require individual strategies and adjustments to the environment to allow for their sensory differences. My aspirations for all the sensory work that I have undertaken with autistic children has been for them to gain an understanding of their sensory issues, find strategies to manage these difficulties and be able to cope successfully with everyday situations.

When I first wrote this book in 2008, it explored sensory differences in autistic children, but these differences were not incorporated in the diagnostic criteria for autism. It was not until 2013 that sensory was included in the DSM-5 diagnostic criteria. Since the first edition of my book, there has been more research on sensory issues and autism but there is still a long way to go to fully understand this complex area.

Sensory experiences are perceived differently by everyone. Through the book, I have included quotes from autistic individuals describing their sensory experiences, descriptions from my observations of autistic children and descriptions from parents and carers about their child. I hope these will give you an insight into the sensory world of the autistic child and help you to support the child.

This resource has been developed from an action research project that aimed to explore and enhance understanding of the sensory differences exhibited by children with autism. I investigated the prevalence of sensory differences exhibited in a group of children with autism attending a special school and considered how sensory processing in autistic children impacted on their ability to access the learning environment and on their behaviour. Since then, I have taught and supported many more children displaying sensory differences and continued to develop supportive environments and activities. There had been a rapid rise in the number of children with autism attending the school. Some of the children in the school often appeared to be in a 'world of their own' and had difficulty using their senses to explore their environment; others would become distressed in certain environments or activities. I read lots of the research into sensory processing that was available at the time and the written accounts of autistic adults describing their experiences. At the start of the research project, parents and practitioners completed a Sensory Questionnaire on the children and the results were analysed. Leekam et al. (2007) found that more than 90% of autistic children had sensory difficulties, and the results from the sensory questionnaires showed the same correlation and indicated a high prevalence of significant sensory difficulties. Analysis of the Sensory Questionnaire showed reactions to sensory stimuli that resulted in behaviours that caused significant difficulties for the child both at home and school.

As a staff team, we looked at the environment through a 'sensory lens' to try to identify possible causes for the children's difficulties and thought about changes that we could put in place. A variety of calming spaces were created around the building. More sensory resources were purchased to increase the amount of multisensory experiences we could provide in the curriculum and we planned sensory activities designed to support the individual's needs. The development of a multisensory soft play room enabled the room to be turned into a themed area that was linked to curriculum modules. This was an exciting development, as it enabled the creation of an environment for dance, drama, music and role play which focused on sensory experiences. The outside environment was also developed to enrich the children's play opportunities and the use of a sensory garden allowed more sensory exploratory work to take place.

Parents and carers have considerable insight into their children, and their input into building a sensory profile of their child made an invaluable contribution to the knowledge gained. Parents described a high prevalence of unusual reactions to stimuli, with children having difficulties in several sensory areas. However, it is the severity of the response to a stimulus that determines whether the child's reaction is a problem or not. For example, parents often report difficulties getting children to allow the hairdresser to cut their hair or let the parent cut their fingernails. This is the case with many young children; however, for those that are hypersensitive to touch, their response to the situation could be extreme, with the child being terrified and their reaction being to scream for a long period of time, or to bite or kick. As Voss points out:

> We all have sensory preferences and sensory differences. At times, however there are so many sensory differences that it impacts one or more areas of development and quality of life.
> Voss (2015, p113)

A positive outcome of the research was that results from the study highlighted to staff the possible link between behaviour and sensory difficulties for autistic children. This greater awareness of the child's sensory differences led to a better understanding of the possible causes of the child's behaviour. Questionnaire results also indicated that sensory difficulties became more apparent in stressful situations; hence the need for careful consideration of environmental issues.

An interesting finding was that parents, carers and staff reported changes in response to stimuli over time. This raises the question that autistic individuals may be able to cope better with sensory stimuli as they get older, either due to the maturation of the sensory system or because they are employing a strategy that enables them to cope. One parent described how her child reverts back to a particular behaviour when stressed:

> when younger he would lay on the floor and watch wheels of objects. He plays differently now but will revert to this when in a stressful situation.

It was clear from the results of the questionnaires that children had different sensory issues, emphasising the importance for individual adaptations and strategies. Kranowitz's (2003) description of the child as being 'out of sync' seems a very apt description for autistic children, as results indicated an imbalance of sensory input for many of the children in the study. Traditionally, the education of young children has recognised the importance of providing a wide range of experiences and activities to encourage children to explore using their senses. My study leads me to conclude that, for teachers of autistic children, the inclusion of sensory experiences continues to be a priority beyond the Early Years Foundation Stage and should be included in curriculum planning even when children are in National Curriculum, Key Stage One and Two.

With the increase in children being diagnosed with autism and the majority of these children educated in a mainstream setting, this resource is invaluable in highlighting for practitioners the impact that sensory differences can have for autistic children and help them create an autism-friendly environment and strategies to support the child's sensory needs. This resource, although designed for autistic children, would also be helpful for any child who has sensory difficulties.

This book has not been written to replace the valuable work that occupational therapists do. As Koscinski says:

> the slogan for occupational therapy has become 'skills for the job of living'.
> Koscinki (2016, p16)

However, not everyone can access an assessment and advice from an occupational therapist when it is needed, and I hope this book will increase understanding and give some helpful strategies to help the child cope in day-to-day situations.

If you have not been able to understand the reason for an autistic child's unusual behaviour, been surprised at their reaction to what you have considered to be an irrelevant sensory stimulus or found some of the child's behaviour challenging, then by reading this book, I hope you will gain a greater understanding of sensory differences and will reconsider their behaviour through a sensory lens.

As Voss (2015) points out:

> Understanding a child's sensory needs and differences can truly change the quality of life for that child.
> Voss (2015, p114)

References

Koscinki, C. (2016), *The Parent's Guide to Occupational Therapy for Autism and Other Special Needs*, London: Jessica Kingsley Publishers.

Kranowitz, C. (2003), *The Out of Sync Child Has Fun: Activities for Kids with Sensory Integration Dysfunction*, New York: Berkley Publishing Group.

Leekam, S., Carmen, N., Libby, S., Wing, L., and Gould, J. (2007), Describing the Sensory Abnormalities of Children and Adults with Autism, *Autism Development Disorder* 37: 894–910.

Voss, A. (2015), *Understanding Your Child's Sensory Signals*, ebook.

1 | Understanding autism

It is important to consider the language we use when we talk about autism, as it can affect attitudes. In the past, having a diagnosis of autism has often had negative connotations. This is changing as more research has been undertaken and autobiographical works by autistic individuals and those who have a diagnosis of Asperger syndrome have been published. Many people who have a diagnosis of autism do not think they are disabled but describe it as having a different way of thinking and perceiving the world.

> My autism means I am differently abled! I'm pleased we are not all the same and that I can contribute in a way that someone else might not.
> Lawson (2008, p98)

I believe it is important to give a positive message about autism, recognising and celebrating an individual's strengths but also understanding the differences and possible challenges the individual with autism might face.

Brugha et al. (2012) found that around 700,000 people may have autism, or more than 1 in 100 in the population. The National Autistic Society (2020) estimates that autism is three times more prevalent in boys than in girls although it is now thought that many girls go undiagnosed. This could partly be due to the diagnostic criteria focusing on male behaviour and traits. However, recently increasing numbers of girls have been receiving an autism diagnosis. Autistic girls present differently, often being shy or passive, having an increased ability to copy the behaviour of their peers to fit in and their intense interests often focusing on similar things to other girls.

Vermeulen (2001) believes that autistic people process information and think differently from people without autism and states:

> The essence of autism does not lie in external behaviour and is not outwardly visible. It is a problem of being able to assign meaning to things. This is a problem shared by all persons with autism, yet the way in which this problem manifests itself (in behavioural terms) varies enormously.
> Vermeulen (2001, p14)

He believes that to gain a better understanding of autistic behaviour, you need to get 'inside' the brain of an autistic person and discover how the individual 'processes external auditory, visual and physical experiences' Vermeulen (2001, p14).

Traditionally, both in the diagnostic criteria and in educational settings, an individual is assessed by what they 'can't do'. All of us would fall short if we were solely judged by our deficits. Many of the ways that autistic individuals make sense of the world can be viewed in terms of a strength, if we consider what is often described as the individual's problem making sense of the situation or not seeing the 'big picture'. We can flip that to describe their superior ability to have detailed focus. Many autistic individuals are extremely good at focusing on detail. There are many careers that require great accuracy and the ability for the person to look at fine detail. Many autistic people are particularly suited to these types of careers and all businesses would benefit from having a worker that ensures all the details of a project are correct and spots errors and inconsistencies.

Some individuals have incredible abilities and are described as autistic savants. One young person I know is able to say what day of the week you were born when he is given your birth date; another adult, who is now 33 years old, can remember each birthday present he received from the age of 3. Stephen Wiltshire, MBE, is an artist who draws very detailed cityscapes. He has an amazing eye for detail and can draw from memory a landscape after seeing it just once. Autistic individuals can often focus on their special interest for extended periods of time and become very knowledgeable about the subject. This ability to focus has led to many advances in science and technology.

As Lawrence points out:

> Those who have the most heightened sensory acuity are revered by society – the top perfumiers, the chocolatier, the musician who hears the finest nuances of a piece or the conductor who follows each part within a symphony.
> Lawrence (2019, p19)

The autistic person has an individual way of looking at the world – sometimes referred to as 'thinking outside the box'. We are all unique and although autistic individuals share certain features it affects everyone differently. You cannot always tell if someone is autistic from their appearance and it is often referred to as a hidden disability.

Autism was recognised by Leo Kanner in 1943. He believed that autism resulted from problems occurring in the developing brain. His work (Kanner 1943) described the case histories of 11 children who had in common an unusual pattern of behaviour. Kanner described them as having:

• Difficulty with social relationships

• Difficulty with social communication

• Rigidity of thought and impaired imagination

These were referred to as 'The Triad of Impairments' (Wing, 2002), and Kanner's criteria were used to diagnose autism. There have been many terms used to describe autism. Sometimes it is referred to as an autistic spectrum disorder, abbreviated to ASD, or autistic spectrum condition, abbreviated to ASC.

There is currently no medical test that tells you if a child has autism. To get a diagnosis a paediatrician or multidisciplinary team assess the child through a variety of ways – observing the child in different settings, talking to the child, talking to parents about their child's development and behaviour, reports from educational settings.

Recently the two main diagnostic organisations: – the World Health Organisation's (1995) Criteria for Childhood Autism *International Classification of Diseases*, known as **ICD**, and the American Psychiatric Association's *Diagnostic and Statistical Manual of Mental Disorders*, referred to as **DSM**, have updated their criteria used for diagnosis.

The latest version of **DSM-5** was published in 2013, and the **ICD-11** was released in 2018. Both organisations describe the characteristics of autism as difficulties in interaction and social communication on the one hand, and restricted interests and repetitive behaviours on the other.

The DSM-5 includes autism within the neurodevelopmental disorders category. In the DSM-5 diagnostic criteria, the emphasis is on identifying an individual's needs and how much their autism affects their ability to function in everyday life.

A separate diagnosis of Asperger syndrome is no longer given and is included under the umbrella term 'autistic spectrum' in the diagnostic criteria. Many people strongly identify with their diagnosis of Asperger syndrome and do not approve of Asperger syndrome not being a separate condition. However, if an individual had already been given Asperger syndrome as a diagnosis they can keep the label.

Wing (2002) describes Asperger syndrome as often being associated with the more able children on the spectrum. The child is likely to be more verbal but still have difficulties with social interaction. The condition was described by Hans Asperger in 1944. He had a very positive attitude towards those who have the syndrome and wrote:

> it seems that for success in science or art a dash of autism is essential. For success the necessary ingredient may be an ability to turn from the everyday world, from the simply practical, an ability to rethink a subject with originality so as to create untrodden ways, with all abilities channelled into the one speciality.
> Asperger, H. (1979) Problems of infantile autism cited in Attwood (2005, p126)

The DSM-5, the diagnostic criteria are described as

A. Persistent deficits in social communication and social interaction across multiple contexts

1 Deficits in social-emotional reciprocity

The child, for example, may have good language skills but has difficulty taking turns in a conversation and talks about their own special interest for a long time, with no regard to whether the listener is paying attention or is interested. Others may not speak or have limited speech. The child may be echolalic, repeating what someone else has said. The child may not initiate or respond to social interactions. They may have difficulty recognising their own and others' emotions. The child's ability to understand other people's feelings and understand the reason behind other people's actions or intentions can be affected. They may approach others in an inappropriate physical or verbal manner, misreading subtle social cues and behaviours in others. For some children, anxiety affects their behaviour and thoughts every day, interfering with their school, home and social life.

2 Deficits in nonverbal communicative behaviours used for social interaction

The child may have difficulty understanding gesture, body language, tone of voice and facial expression. They may take things literally and not understand jokes or sarcasm.

3 Deficits in developing, maintaining and understanding relationships

The child may have difficulty adjusting their behaviour to suit different social situations. The child may appear to be in a world of their own and not seek out others to share an experience. Others may want friends but do not seem to understand how to do this and find it hard to form friendships.

B. Restricted, repetitive patterns of behaviour, interests or activities, as manifested by at least two of the following, currently or in the past

1 Stereotyped or repetitive motor movements or use of objects or speech

The child may, for example, line up toys, repeat actions such as rocking, spinning themselves or objects, making repetitive sounds or repeating phrases.

2 Insistence on sameness, inflexible adherence to routines, or ritualised patterns or verbal nonverbal behaviour

The child likes routine and things to be predictable, and may get extremely distressed at small changes and find transitions very difficult to cope with. They have a rigid thinking pattern which can result in the child being inflexible and unwilling to change their ideas or behaviour when circumstances change. They may have problems with organising and planning tasks and activities.

3 Highly restricted, fixated interests that are abnormal in intensity or focus

The child may have an intense interest and may be preoccupied with unusual objects or interests. Sometimes the special interest can become all consuming, with the child thinking about it from the time they wake up to the time they go to sleep, having difficulty focusing on anything else.

4 Hyper- or hyporeactivity to sensory input or unusual interests in sensory aspects of the environment

The child may experience too much sensory input which may, for example, cause an adverse response or they may not recognise a sensory input and may not react. They may be fascinated by a sensory stimulus and for example, like to watch moving lights, spinning wheels or fans.

Leo Kanner, in his 1943 paper 'Autistic Disturbances of Affective Contact', noticed and described reactivity to sensory input with the children he observed.

His description of a boy called Donald describes how he made

> stereotyped movements with his fingers, crossing them about in the air. He shook his head from side to side, whispering or humming the same three note tune. He spun with great pleasure anything he could seize upon to spin.
> Kanner (1943, p219)

Autistic individuals have described their sensory differences ever since Kanner's original description of autism. Although the inclusion of hypersensitivity and hyposensitivity was proposed for the DSM-3 diagnostic criteria which was published in 1980, it was not included as it was not considered to be an 'essential feature'. Wing (1996), referring to behaviours and responses to sensory stimulation, states that:

> these behaviours are common but by no means universal and are not crucial to diagnosis.
> Wing (1996, p48)

I agree that no two people with autism exhibit the same behavioural profile, but the more I worked with autistic children, the more I questioned the relevance of the way they interpreted sensory experiences and its relationship to behaviour. However, it was not until 2013 in the DSM-5 that sensory difficulties were included in the diagnostic criteria. The inclusion of sensory difficulties in the diagnosis has been welcomed, as many autistic people feel they can be more debilitating than issues related to social interaction and communication. As Casanova writing in Bogdashina (2016, p11) explains, 'sensory problems are with you every minute of every day. In effect, sensory disorders colour all aspects of your life experiences'.

Heffernan (2016) says that:

> a very significant step on the path to understanding the autistic perspective has been the burgeoning recognition of the part sensory issues play in the lives of people with autism. Heffernan (2016, p11)

In the next chapter, we will look in more detail at sensory processing and how sensory differences can impact on the individual.

References

American Psychiatric Association. (2013) *Diagnostic and Statistical Manual of Mental Disorders, Fifth Edition (DSM-5)*, United States of America: American Psychiatric Association.

Attwood, T. (2005), *Asperger's Syndrome*, London: Jessica Kingsley Publishers.

Brugha, T. et al. (2012). *Estimating the Prevalence of Autism Spectrum Conditions in Adults: Extending the 2007 Adult Psychiatric Morbidity Survey*, Leeds: NHS Information Centre for Health and Social Care.

Cassanova, M., writing in Bogdashina, O. (2016), *Sensory Perceptual Issues in Autism and Asperger Syndrome, Second Edition: Different Sensory Experiences – Different Perceptual Worlds*, London: Jessica Kingsley Publishers.

Heffernan, D. (2016), *Sensory Issues for Adults with Autism Spectrum Disorder*, London: Jessica Kingsley Publishers.

Kanner, L. (1943), Autistic Disturbances of Affective Contact, *Nervous Child* 2: 217–250.

Lawrence, C. (2019), *Teacher Education and Autism*, London: Jessica Kingsley Publishers.

Lawson, W. (2008), *Concepts of Normality- The Autistic and Typical Syndrome*, London: Jessica Kingsley Publishers.

National Autistic Society. (2020), website https://www.autism.org.uk/about/what-is/gender.aspx

Vermeulen, P. (2001), *Autistic Thinking, This Is the Title*, London: Jessica Kingsley.

Wing, L. (1996), *The Autistic Spectrum*, London: Constable and Robinson.

World Health Organisation (1995), *International Classification of Diseases and Related Health Problems* (ICD 10), World Health Organisation.

2 | Sensory differences and autism

Recently there have been many published accounts written by autistic people in which they describe their experiences and give us a greater insight into the problems they encounter.

We all have sensory preferences and dislikes; for example, some people love intense flavours like Marmite, whilst others hate it. For some people, however, their sensory experiences create significant problems that interfere with their ability to function. Lawson (2000), who has a diagnosis of autistic spectrum disorder, encounters and processes sensory experiences differently.

> What I do realise is that I do not see the world as others do. Most people take the routines of life and day-to-day connections for granted. The fact they can see, hear, smell, touch and relate to others is 'normal'. For me, these things are often painfully overwhelming, non-existent or just confusing.
> Lawson (2000, p2)

Other researchers have also recognised the impact of sensory difficulties. Scott, cited in Ariel and Naseef, states:

> the ranges of heightened or reduced sensory processing in all areas, smell, sight, hearing, touch, and taste - that are seen in individuals with an autistic spectrum disorder should not be underestimated. It is most likely that behaviours seen by us as inexplicable and bizarre are in fact reactions to stimuli that are, for them extreme.
> Scott cited in Ariel and Naseef (2006, p258)

Sensory systems and how we process information

We find out about the world through our senses. We are all exceptional in the way that we perceive the world. Our perception of the world is unique, and it can result in us having a different response to others that are experiencing the same sensory information. Understanding the way our sensory systems work is very complex and greater research needs to be done on the subject.

> When we understand how our sensory systems work, we can better understand why we do the things we do or act the way we do. In short our sensory systems help us 'make sense' of the world.
> Smith Myles et al. (2000, p18)

When people refer to the senses, they often only think of five senses.

- **Touch or tactile system:** Receptors in the skin enable us to feel textures, the temperature of objects, pressure and pain.

- **Sight or visual system:** Receptors in the retina of the eye enable us to distinguish objects, colours and spatial awareness.

- **Sound or auditory system:** Receptors in the inner ear enable us to hear sounds in the environment.

- **Taste or gustatory system:** Receptors in the tongue enable us to distinguish between sweet, sour, bitter and salty.

- **Smell or olfactory system:** Receptors in the nose enable us to distinguish smells.

There are three other sensory systems which are also important for our understanding of the world.

- **Vestibular system:** Receptors are situated in the inner ear. The fluid in the ear enables us to know the position of our head and body. It gives us information on direction and movement. This enables us to keep our balance and posture.

- **Proprioceptive system:** Receptors are situated in our joints and muscles. They enable us to know our body position in relation to objects and other people. The proprioceptive system also gives us information on the amount of force needed to complete an activity; for example, the system provides information on how much effort is needed to pick up a heavy object like a chair or a light object like a feather. The proprioceptive system helps us to co-ordinate our movements.

- **Interoception:** Receptors are situated all over our body, including in the organs of the body, the skin and bones. These give the brain information about the inside of your body. The sense of interoception allows us to feel what is happening inside our body. For example, it tells us if we are thirsty or hungry, if we have eaten enough, whether we are too hot or too cold, and if we are feeling ill.

Neuroscientists are now able to scan the brain using imaging techniques and they are continually discovering more details about the complex working of the brain. The brain is constantly receiving and processing information from the sensory systems. Sensory stimuli changes into electrical signals and these are sent to the central nervous system, which is made up of the spinal cord and brain, through an interconnecting network of nerve cells.

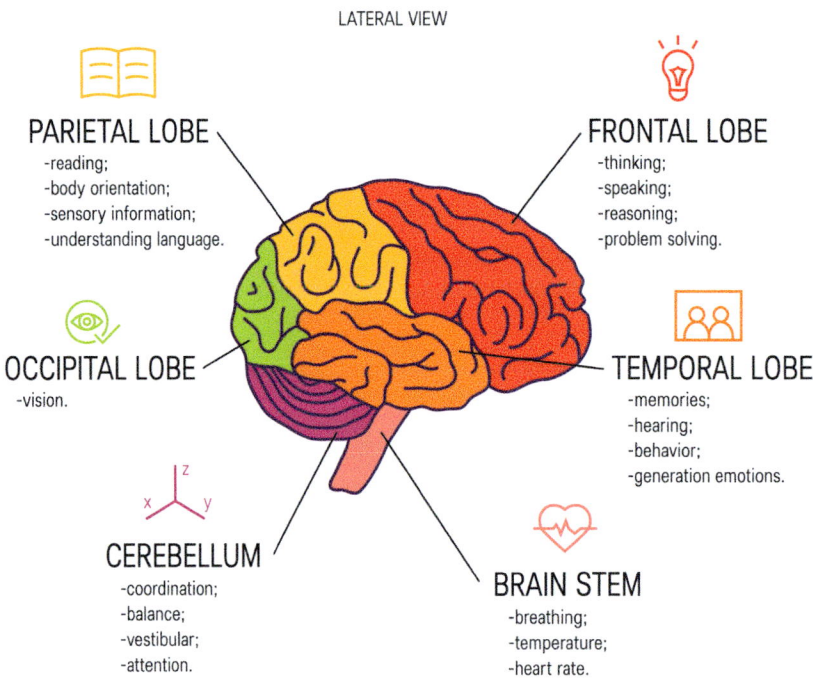

FUNCTIONAL AREAS OF THE BRAIN

LATERAL VIEW

PARIETAL LOBE
-reading;
-body orientation;
-sensory information;
-understanding language.

FRONTAL LOBE
-thinking;
-speaking;
-reasoning;
-problem solving.

OCCIPITAL LOBE
-vision.

TEMPORAL LOBE
-memories;
-hearing;
-behavior;
-generation emotions.

CEREBELLUM
-coordination;
-balance;
-vestibular;
-attention.

BRAIN STEM
-breathing;
-temperature;
-heart rate.

There are billions of nerve cells called neurons and as we learn, stronger and more direct pathways are developed between them. Whilst when we first learn something, it takes a long time, as the neurons are stimulated repeatedly, electrical signals travel faster and there is an increase in the child's ability to learn. The main part of the brain is the cerebrum which is divided into two parts or hemispheres.

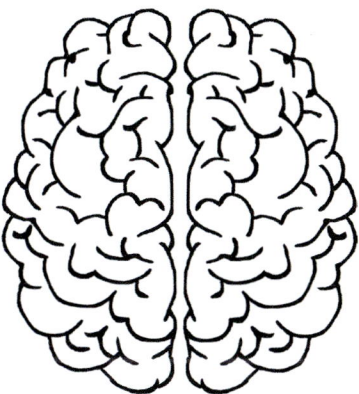

These are connected and information passes between them. Messages from each sensory system are processed in specialised parts of the brain and Longhorn (2000) states that the optimum amount of learning takes place when both hemispheres function effectively together. The cerebellum lies behind the cerebrum and combines information from the ears, eyes and muscles to help co-ordinate movement. The brain stem controls reflexes such as moving away from pain and automatic functions such as heart rate. Its role is to protect the body, and in times of stress, adrenalin levels rise which can block electrical signals from the sensory systems reaching the brain, resulting in the body triggering what is often described as a 'fight or flight' response. As Boucher (2017, p136) points out, 'the brains of many people with autism are in most respects operating effectively, though probably differently from the brains of people without autism'.

Perception

The collection, organisation, interpretation and comprehension of the information coming from our sensory systems is called perception (Bogdashina, 2016). As babies develop, they learn how to make meaning of the information from their senses through interaction with the environment.

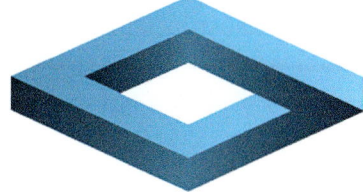

Experience tells us that this drawing is an impossible image.

Our brain is constantly receiving information from different senses and when we are able to interpret the information using the memory and knowledge gained through experiencing the world we can then act appropriately in that situation.

For example, Larkey describes Sensory integration as

> the organisation and processing of sensations from different sensory channels for meaningful use.
> Larkey (2007, p11)

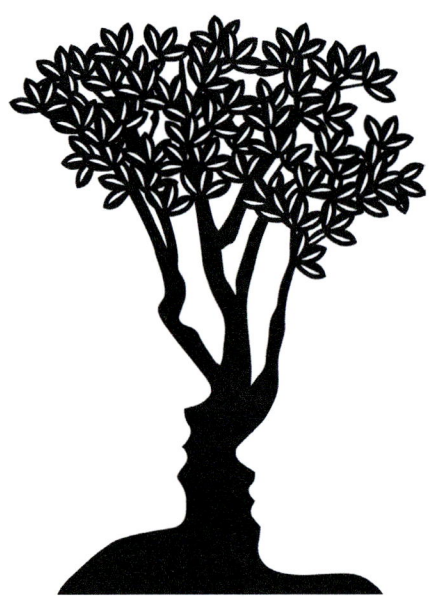

What do you see?

Did you see the tree first or the two faces?

This is an illustration of figure ground perception, where a picture is simplified into a main object, which is called the 'figure', and the background, which is called the 'ground'. Some people will have seen the black tree first, others the white faces. It depends if you saw the black tree as the figure and the white as the ground or vice versa. Most people are able to switch their perception between the two images, seeing first one and then the other.

We often do not perceive a sensory input if it is constantly there; for example, when we enter the kitchen, we may notice the humming sound of the fridge but after a while, we may no longer be aware of it. Attention also affects how we perceive things. If we are intensely interested in something – for example, when talking to a friend in a busy place – we can tune out background noise. Motivation also affects our perception and enables us to identify a sensory stimulus we are interested in when it is embedded in a distracting background.

Sensory issues associated with autism

Lawrence explains that for autistic children,

> different perceptions of the sensory world may be experienced all the time.
> Lawrence (2019, p18)

Wilkes asks us to:

> Imagine what happens when just one or all of the senses are intensified or are not present at all. This difficulty is often called sensory integration dysfunction and it is one that many individuals on the autistic spectrum experience.
> Wilkes (2005, p1)

Sensory integration dysfunction is a term that describes difficulty with processing input from the sensory systems. As Emmons and McKendry Anderson (2005) point out, if the systems do not work 'simultaneously and cooperatively', sensory dysfunction may result. They explain that the term 'sensory integration dysfunction' is often used interchangeably with those of 'sensory dysfunction' and 'sensory processing disorder'. The condition is usually diagnosed by an occupational therapist working with an observational checklist of specific indicators through the observation of children's behaviour.

Autistic children may experience a range of sensory differences:

Hyperreactivity: Many autistic children may be overly sensitive to certain sensations (hypersensitive), resulting in too much stimulation reaching the brain. The child may be unable to ignore this information and may have an extreme reaction. As a coping strategy, they may try to avoid the sensory input.

Hyporeactivity: The child may have low sensitivity (hyposensitive) whereby too little stimulation reaches the brain, and they may not register the sensory stimuli or take longer to respond to it.

Unusual interests in sensory aspects of the environment:

Trying to work out the reason for a particular behaviour is very complex as both hyperreactivity and hyporeactivity can result in sensory-seeking behaviour which means the same behaviour can be caused for different reasons. As Boucher (2017) explains, autistic people often use repetitive sensory behaviours to mitigate overstimulation or compensate for understimulation.

The child who is hyporeactive may be sensory seeking and crave intense sensory experiences to help them make sense of the environment. However, hypersensitivity to a stimulus can also result in the child being fascinated with it (Bogdashina, 2016) and getting intense pleasure from the sensory-seeking behaviour. This is the opposite of being upset by the stimulus and it causes pain or overload. As Fletcher-Watson and Happé (2019) point out, sensory sensitivities can be beneficial and

> many autistic people describe the intense beauty and pleasure of their heightened responses.
> Fletcher-Watson and Happé (2019, p39)

Fascination with certain stimuli can be positive and result in an enjoyable pastime. It also often calms the person with autism. In the same way that I enjoy looking at a panoramic view and may spend a considerable amount of time doing this, for example, I suggest that it is equally valuable for the autistic person, for example, to look at the patterns created by sunlight falling on dust particles or watching a moving fan. Accepting difference is an important element in developing respect for the individual. It is, however, important to bear in mind that fascination with a stimulus can lead to the child withdrawing from what is going on around them. This was the case with one child, who gained intense pleasure from blowing on a feather or any light object and watching it float and sink, repeating this activity continually. However, this repetitive behaviour resulted in staff having difficulty engaging the child in any classroom activity that did not involve visual stimulation – and therefore the self-stimulating behaviour restricted his exploration of the environment.

Sensory differences that can affect any of the senses

Touch

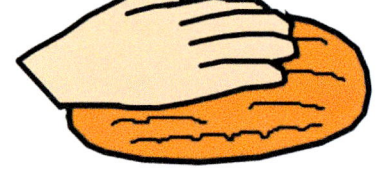

touch

Hyperreactivity, whereby the child is oversensitive to touch, can result in the following:

• Light touch is painful – the child may violently react if someone brushes past and only gently touches them

• Dislikes having anything on hands or feet – the child takes off shoes and socks immediately on entering the room

• Does not like touching a range of different textures

• Avoids putting hands in messy substances

• Does not like wearing certain textures of clothes, irritated by labels in clothes

Wiley (2005) describes ripping the tags out of her clothing and Lawson (2001) also describes this difficulty:

> I only wear cotton next to my skin because of the discomfort with how other materials feel. Lawson (2001, p181)

A parent, whose child was very sensitive to different textures, reported that she had tremendous difficulty getting her child to wear new clothes when the old ones had become too small and that she resorted to buying lots of the same item of clothing in different sizes.

Hyporeactivity, whereby the child is undersensitive to the sense of touch, can result in the following:

• Has a delayed response to textures or touch and needs extra time to process tactile information

• Has a decreased awareness of pain

Unusual interests in tactile sensory aspects of the environment:
The child may display sensory-seeking behaviour which can result in the following behaviours:

• Craves tactile stimulation

• Self-injury; for example, a child may bite themselves or bang their head on the ground – one parent described how their child bit themselves so severely that he often broke the surface of the skin and head butted the floor or walls which has on occasion resulted in severe bruising and hospital treatment

• Seeks very firm hugs

• Frequently touching objects: the child may have a routine for touching items in a room

• Fascination by certain textures and loves to touch them

Sight

Hyperreactivity, whereby the child is oversensitive to the sense of sight, can result in the following:

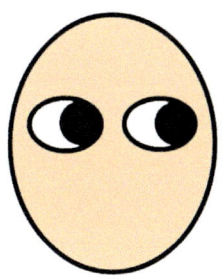

looking

- Does not like certain colours

- Avoids direct eye contact

- Uses peripheral vision (looks at things out of the corner of the eye)

- Hits, rubs eyes when distressed

- Overly sensitive to bright lights

The child may become distressed and cover their eyes when the lights are turned on:

> bright lights, midday sun, reflected lights strobe lights, flickering lights, fluorescent lights; each seemed to sear my eyes.
> Wiley (2005, p26)

A parent described how her toddler only wanted to play outside on dreary, rainy days and it was not until he was given sunglasses and then wanted to play outside all the time that she realised how sensitive he was to sunlight.

The child may be very aware of the slightest change in the environment. One parent described the way the child used his visual sense as seeming to

> scan over things, sometimes seeing shapes or planes in the sky hardly visible to the naked eye. He will comment on things that have altered only very slightly – a radio that has been moved for dusting and I thought put back in the same place.
> quote from parent/carer questionnaire

Hyporeactivity, whereby the child is undersensitive to the sense of sight, can result in the following:

- Appears unaware of contrasting colours

- Appears not to notice obstacles

Unusual interests in visual sensory aspects of the environment:
The child may display sensory-seeking behaviour which can result in the following behaviours:

- Looking intently at people and objects

- Moves head very close to objects to look at them

- Moves fingers in front of eyes to increase stimulation

- Fascination with reflections

- Fascination with brightly coloured objects, moving patterns and colours

One of the children I worked with spent a long time spinning the wheels on their tricycle and watching them. Lawson describes this fascination with spinning wheels and the feelings the activity evoked:

> I turned my new bicycle upside down and spun the wheels, round and round and round. The light gleaming from the silver mudguards seemed to go on forever. It was so intoxicating and I felt so alive. To have that feeling interrupted by so much as a word or an action evoked extreme irritation and anger in me. I hated being disturbed or interrupted when I was involved with some repetitive action that gave me delight. I felt a sense of connection as I watched the shiny mudguards. I felt safe, almost as if I were part of the bike.
> Lawson (2000, p2)

Sound

Hyperreactivity, whereby the child is oversensitive to the sense of hearing, can result in the following:

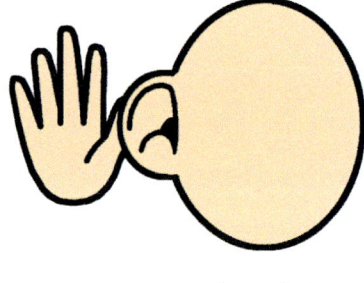

hearing

- Hears sounds in the distance that others cannot hear; one of the children I worked with was able to hear an approaching aeroplane a long time before anyone else and the hum of the fridge in another room which nobody else noticed

- Covers ears to block out sound

- Screams in response to a particular sound, such as the sound of a hand dryer

- Makes repetitive noises to block out sounds they find distressing

- Dislikes noisy places

Grandin, who has autism, explains her inability to cut out particular sounds:

> When two people are talking at once, it is difficult for me to screen out one voice and listen to the other. My ears are like microphones picking up all sounds with equal intensity. Most people's ears are like highly directional microphones, which only pick up sounds from the person they are pointed at. In a noisy place, I can't understand speech, because I cannot screen out background noise. When I was a child, large noisy gatherings of relatives were overwhelming and I would just lose control and throw temper tantrums.
> Grandin (1996, p68)

She also describes that as a child, loud noises felt like a dentist's drill hitting a nerve and actually causing her pain.

Hyporeactivity, whereby the child is undersensitive to the sense of hearing, can result in the following:

- Not acknowledging certain sounds

- Having a delayed response to a sound or verbal information or instruction, and needing extra time to process information

A delay in responding to speech can create difficulties for the child as people often do not allow enough time for the child to process spoken language. During an observation, I recorded 20 seconds had passed before the child showed any indication that they had heard what had been said, but after this time delay was then able to follow the instruction.

Unusual interests in auditory sensory aspects of the environment:
The child may display sensory-seeking behaviour which can result in the following behaviours:

- Likes sounds to be repeated – bangs doors or objects continually, turns the TV on and off, replays TV clips

- Puts ear close to a sound to listen

- Enjoys loud noises

- Frequently makes repetitive noises, e.g. humming, clicking sounds, chants favourite words

- Fascination with certain sounds

Taste

Hyperreactivity, whereby the child is oversensitive to the sense of taste, can result in the following:

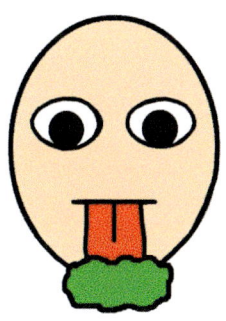

tasting

- A restricted diet as a result of their taste buds being oversensitive

- Gags when eating certain foods

- Certain textures of food cause discomfort

- Does not like trying new foods

- Shows extreme reaction when cleaning teeth

Hypersensitivity to taste can cause considerable anxiety for parents, due to the serious – and indeed, possibly life-threatening – implications of the very restricted diets that many children follow. Many parents express concern over their children's diets. This can be illustrated by one child who attended the school, whose diet for over four years consisted of Fromage Frais, chocolate buttons and orange squash. Parents also described how their children would accept a particular food for a period of time and then refuse to eat it. Some children could only tolerate crunchy food, whilst others only ate soft foods.

Hyporeactivity, whereby the child is undersensitive to the sense of taste, can result in the following:

- Eating any food presented to them

- Showing no preferences for particular tastes

Unusual interests in gustatory sensory aspects of the environment:
The child may display sensory-seeking behaviour which can result in the following behaviours:

- Craves certain foods

- Licks or bites objects or people – one school year I do not think we had a single toy in the classroom that had not got bite marks in it as one child explored his environment by putting everything into his mouth

- Likes chewing on things for long time

- Chews non-edible objects – one child continually sought inedible substances to eat or lick and would eat glue, paper, plastic toys, play dough and Blu Tack; one day at snack time he took the raisins out of the cardboard box and proceeded to eat the box (a craving for things that have no nutritional value is called Pica). Wiley describes:

  > I loved to chew crunchy things, even if they were poisonous. . . . I shaved the sand off Emery boards with my front teeth. I took great delight in grinding the striking strip of a match book between my front teeth.
  > Wiley (2005, p25)

- Fascination with certain foods

Smell

Hyperreactivity, whereby the child is oversensitive to the sense of smell, can result in the following:

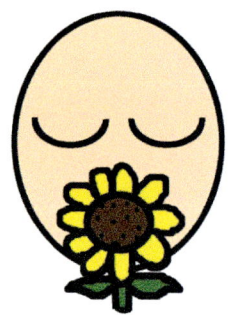

smelling

- Smells that are intensified and become overpowering – the child may dislike adults wearing perfume or dislike the smell of the washing powder on their clothes

- Strong dislike for certain smells which we may think of as pleasant

- Certain smells cause the child to feel nauseous

- Hits nose when distressed

- Gags when smelling certain smells

Hyporeactivity, whereby the child is undersensitive to the sense of smell, can result in the following:

- Does not notice extreme odours

- Has difficulty recognising food smells

Unusual interests in olfactory sensory aspects of the environment:

The child may display sensory-seeking behaviour which can result in the following behaviours:

- The need to smell themselves and others

- Frequently smells objects; one child in the classroom would constantly rub his nose against objects and smell them. When he was reading a book, he would smell it each time he turned the page. He would also smell people when they entered the room. If they stood up from their chair, he would smell where they had been seated. This sensory-seeking behaviour caused a problem when on outings with his family, as many people did not understand this behaviour

- Seeks strong odours

- Smells and plays with faeces

- Fascinated by certain smells

Vestibular

Hyperreactivity, whereby the child is oversensitive to the vestibular sense, can result in the following:

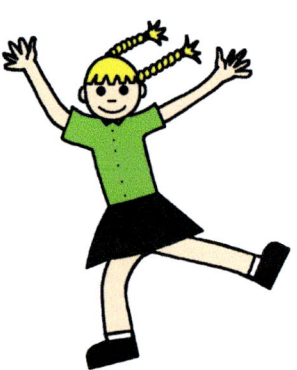

- Frightened of activities in which their feet leave the ground

- Avoids balancing activities

- Dislikes swinging activities

- Dislikes activities involving changes in head position

- Dislikes walking on uneven surfaces

Hyporeactivity, whereby the child is undersensitive to the vestibular sense, can result in the following:

- Does not get dizzy if spins for an extended amount of time

- Appears unaware of risks when climbing or running

Unusual interests in vestibular sensory aspects of the environment:
The child may display sensory-seeking behaviour which can result in the following behaviours:

- Craves rocking or spinning sensations – one of the children in the classroom often laid on the floor and rocked from side to side

- Frequently turning upside down

- Paces up and down

- Unable to sit still, constantly moving

- Craves fast movement – always running rather than walking; Gardner describes her son's running:

> He would charge across the room, bounce himself off the wall to gain momentum and race back again – droning continuously, sometimes in a happy tone, sometimes anxious. This would go on for hours and he never tired. He did this so often the plaster on the walls started to bulge and separate where he bounced off them. . . . If anyone tried to stop him he would respond with a challenging tantrum.
> Gardner (2007, p20)

Proprioception

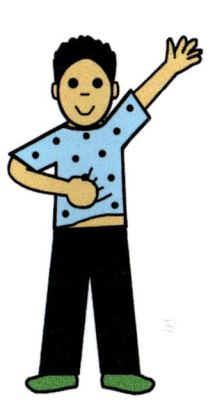

Hyperreactivity, whereby the child is oversensitive to the proprioceptive sense, can result in the following:

- Dislikes certain movements

- Difficulty with fine motor skills

- Dislikes fast-moving activities

- Difficulty with gross motor skills – e.g. catching a ball, climbing a ladder

- Dislikes rough and tumble play

Hyporeactivity, whereby the child is undersensitive to the proprioceptive sense, can result in the following:

- Has difficulty knowing the position of their body – unaware of position of objects and other people and bumps into them

- Unaware of how much force to use when doing a task – e.g. holds a pencil too tightly when writing

Unusual interests in proprioceptive sensory aspects of the environment:
The child may display sensory-seeking behaviour which can result in the following behaviours:

- Likes to be hugged very tightly or squeezed – one parent described how her son likes to be squeezed hard and that she finds this is helpful if he is having a meltdown as it appears to 'release anxiety'

- Seeks rough and tumble play

- Likes to get into small, tight places

- Likes to lean on furniture/against walls

- Fascinated by movement

Interoception

Hyperreactivity, whereby the child is oversensitive to the interoception sense, can result in the following:

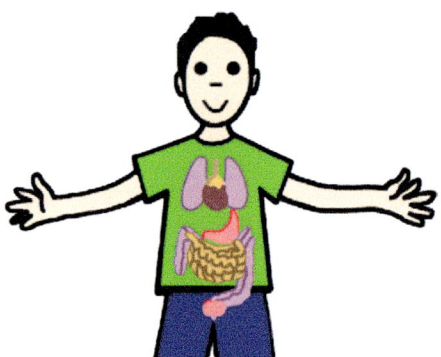

• May feel pain more acutely or for longer periods of time than other people

• May be excessively bothered by a small injury

• May feel hot or cold more intensely than others

• Does not like the sensation of being hungry and may eat excessively to avoid the sensation

• Does not like the sensation of being thirsty and may drink excessively to avoid the sensation

Hyporeactivity, whereby the child is undersensitive to the interoception sense and may have a reduced awareness of body sensations, which can result in the following:

• May not recognise they are hungry or thirsty, too hot or too cold

• May not recognise they are ill

• May be aware that something is wrong but be unable to accurately identify where these sensory signals are coming from or recognise what they mean

• May not be aware of pain signals unless they are extremely intense

As the feeling of pain is the body's way of warning us of danger and if this response is lacking, there could be a link between the decreased awareness of pain and the fearless behaviour described by parents, carers and educational practitioners. Parents reported that the children may, for example, climb on furniture, out of windows, or to the top of trees without any fear. One child cycled his tricycle into a wall, cutting his head and leg badly, and showed no registration of pain and no sign of discomfort. This could cause a major difficulty for the child as they may not be aware that they have hurt themselves and therefore not react appropriately in a potentially dangerous situation. Many parents have reported not recognising the severity of their child's injury following an accident as the child had not cried or sought comfort. This also has implications for staffing at school, as in order to keep the children safe, a high level of staffing is necessary.

Fiene and Brownlow's (2015) research found that autistic adults had a significantly deceased awareness of interoception. However, there has been relatively little research into interoception and its impact on autistic individuals.

Unusual interests in interoceptive sensory aspects of the environment:
The child may display sensory-seeking behaviour which can result in the following behaviours:

• May eat excessively

• May drink excessively

• Fascinated by internal bodily sensations

Other sensory differences which can cause difficulties for the child

Being hyperreactive and hyporeactive within the same sensory system

Some children may be both hyperreactive and hyporeactive in the same sensory system, depending on the stimulus. One child was both hypersensitive and hyposensitive to tactile input. He found different textures of clothing difficult to tolerate and he would scream when asked to put on a new coat or jumper. However, he also had a decreased awareness of pain. The parent reported the child

> reacts as if some clothing is actually causing pain. He will however, lean on very hot radiators and not notice they are so very hot.
> quote from parent/carer questionnaire

Another child did not show any response to a loud bang directly behind them but the same child found the fan on the heater impossible to tolerate, resulting in screaming and the child refusing to enter the room.

Inconsistency of reaction to stimuli

Reactions to sensory stimuli can be inconsistent. As Mahler explains:

> The ability to tolerate sensory experiences fluctuates with a variety of factors including our levels of stress, how much we slept the night before or how predictable the situation is at hand. A young person with autism is no different. When a young person is stressed, sleep deprived or in an unpredictable situation, the ability to tolerate sensory experiences goes down.
> Mahler (2018, p6)

Many children I have worked with often showed different reactions to sensory stimulus, depending on such things as the environment, what demands were being placed on them, if they were feeling tired or hungry, and their stress levels. These factors all affected how efficiently their sensory systems worked. One parent describes how their child

> does not cope well with noises in an adjacent room. He constantly asks for it to be quieter. Everything needs to be 'quieter'. He will listen to radio/CD player at such a low volume it is barely audible.

However, the parent reported that on other occasions he does not respond to a sound or an instruction.

Changes over time

A sensory experience that a young child finds overwhelming may not cause such a difficulty as they get older. Autistic individuals may be able to cope better with sensory stimuli as they get older, either because they are using a strategy that enables them to cope or due to the maturation of the sensory system. One parent described how she helped her child cope in a stressful situation:

> Busy places bother him such as airports and parties. We put headphones on him to block out the background noise and he seems happier.

She also describes how he reverts back to a particular behaviour when stressed. She can always recognise that he is sensory overloaded when he seeks out the headphones.

Modulating a response to stimuli

As sensory information is processed, the child may receive too much stimulation and become overaroused or too little stimulation and be underaroused. When we are aware that we need to calm down or become more active, we may choose a sensory strategy to facilitate or inhibit the sensory message going to the brain. Most of us are able to do this; for example, drinking coffee to become more alert or taking a bath to relax us. Autistic individuals may be unable to modulate their responses and may overreact or underreact to situations.

Differences in perception

When an autistic person is presented with too much information for them to process, they may be unable to interpret their surroundings as a whole picture but only process the parts that attract their attention. This could result in the inability to make meaning from a situation. Bogdashina (2016) describes this as 'fragmented perception'. If sensory information is perceived piece by piece, the autistic person may, for example, not recognise someone if they are wearing unfamiliar clothes or not recognise a place if approached from a different direction.

Isaacs (2015) describes his difficulty making meaning of sensory input:

> I can only process my surroundings one piece at a time, much like a floating jigsaw puzzle. This is also the same with people; I focus on one area and 'lose' another part of them.
> Isaacs writing in Attwood et al. (2015, p23)

Frith (1989) describes the processing style whereby the individual has a focus on detail rather than processing the whole situation as 'weak central coherence'. In the past, this has been referred to as a deficit but the superior performance that many autistic individuals achieve in tasks requiring a focus on detail is now recognised and can be of great value. This was observed in the classroom when the child appeared to pay great attention to small parts of a toy train rather than the whole and was aware of all the minute details. This focus on detail can, however, lead to difficulties interpreting information; for example, one child who was fascinated by moving objects became so absorbed watching the wheels of the cars that he was unable to focus on the whole scene and was not aware of the danger of fast-moving vehicles in the street.

I have noticed that many autistic children often have difficulty perceiving the passage of time and, for example, estimating how long it takes to complete a task.

Autistic individuals are often extremely good at finding details embedded within a busy picture or the environment.

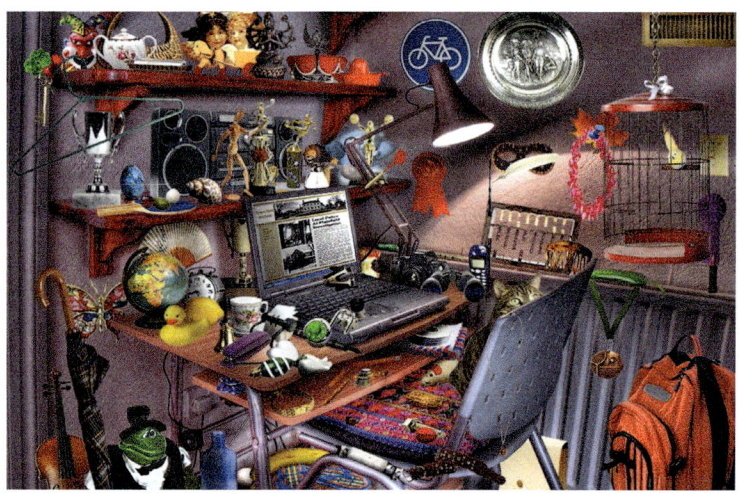

How quickly can you find the lion in the busy picture?

Monotropism

Most people are able to use their senses simultaneously. Lawson (2001) describes 'monotropism' as being able to absorb information from only one sensory channel at a time. A person using 'monotropic thinking' – unlike the neurotypical person, who is able to look at the speaker and listen to what is being said – is able to only focus on one thing and use one sensory channel at a time. Being highly focused on an activity makes it difficult to shift attention from that activity to another.

Filtering sensory information

We take in millions of bits of sensory information each day. Being able to filter out from all the sensory information entering the brain what is important, store what we need for the future and ignore the rest is a vital skill. We are able, for example, to listen and watch a television programme and ignore background sounds but if someone calls 'help' or the fire alarm goes off, we register this information and respond appropriately. Sometimes when entering the perfume department of a shop, we can find the smell intense and overpowering but very quickly our brain is able to block out some of the smell and this prevents us becoming overwhelmed. For many autistic children who have difficulty filtering sensory information, this can quickly lead to sensory overload. Grandin (2006) describes how noises that most people could tune out drove her to distraction.

Sensory differences and a link to social difficulties

Thye et al. (2018) suggest that there is a stronger relationship between sensory difficulties and social interaction than was previously thought. Difficulties processing sensory information could be the cause, or they could exacerbate many of the social difficulties the autistic person experiences. If the autistic individual is unable to filter out background noise and listen to the other person, it can have a negative impact on their ability to socially interact in group situations or busy environments. Being able to process a multitude of sensory stimuli is essential in complex social interactions and helps us to understand other people's body language and social cues and interpret another person's intentions.

Interoception and its link to emotions

Green et al. (2016) found that altered sensory function was associated with emotional problems and restricted repetitive behaviours. The sense of interoception allows us to 'feel' what is going on inside our bodies. Mahler (2018) explains that when we can clearly recognise these signals from our body they become clues to what emotion we are feeling. For example, you can recognise you are scared when you experience sensations such as your heart beating faster, muscles trembling, sweating and your breathing quickening. The interoception system allows us to keep our body in a state of homeostasis, which means it regulates and keeps it stable so that it can function properly. We are able to sense what our body needs and then take action to meet that need. If we recognise that we are thirsty, we are able to meet our body's need and make ourselves feel more comfortable by getting ourselves a drink. If we recognise that we are feeling cold, we can act and get a coat. By taking this action, we are able to self-regulate. The child with interoception difficulties may be aware that something is wrong but be unable to accurately identify where these sensory signals are coming from or recognise what they mean. This can result in them becoming anxious, upset or angry, and they may not be able to say why. This difficulty recognising or understanding your body's internal sensations not only results in difficulty identifying and regulating your emotions, but it will also have an impact on recognising the signs that tell us how another person is feeling. Research (Brewer et al., 2016) indicates an association between interoceptive sensitivity and alexithymia in autistic people. Alexithymia is often described as having 'no words for emotion'. People who have alexithymia often know they are experiencing an emotion but do not know which emotion it is. Later research, (Murphy and Bird, 2018) showed mixed results, and in order to gain a greater understanding of the relationship between alexithymia, autism and interoception, further large scale research is needed.

Sensory overload

Godwin Emmons and McKendry Anderson (2005, p97) assert that it is the sensory issues or needs that drive behaviour and therefore, 'it makes sense to tease apart challenging behaviours using a sensory-based perspective'. Attwood (2015, p97) explains that adults have more opportunities to 'create a lifestyle that minimises the risk of encountering specific unpleasant sensory experiences' than the child. As the child matures, many find strategies to help them cope and find ways to communicate what is troubling them. Young autistic children often cannot do this and can find sensory stimuli extremely intense and quickly become overwhelmed. They may be unable to articulate what is causing them distress and their reaction to the sensory experience may be to display difficult or challenging behaviour.

Sensory overload can cause different reactions; the child may 'shut down' to try to block out the stimulus. The child becomes unable to process sensory information and this can affect one or more senses, resulting in the child being incapable of responding. A parent described how her son would 'shut down' by dropping to the floor and appear to be asleep whenever she entered a noisy environment such as the shopping centre. The child may run away or hide to try to escape from the situation or become verbally or physically aggressive. Some autistic children may communicate their sensory overload by repetitive actions. Grandin (1996) describes how she used the repetitive actions of rocking and spinning as a coping strategy when she became bombarded with stimuli:

> Rocking and spinning were other ways to shut out the outside world when I became so overloaded with too much noise. Rocking made me feel calm. It was like taking an addictive drug. The more I did it the more I wanted to do it.
> Grandin (1996, p44)

People who do not have an understanding of the autistic child's sensory differences may mistakenly interpret a sensory meltdown as the child trying to get what he or she wants, or think they are attention seeking or spoilt. Bogdashina explains that:

> As children are unable to cope with the demands of the world they are not equipped to deal with, they are likely to display behavioural problems, such as self-stimulation, self-injury, aggression, avoidance, rigidity, high anxiety, panic attacks, etc. It is important to remember these children have no control over their problems as they are caused by neurological differences.
> Bogdashina (2005, p215)

As Miller (2010) points out:

> It is easy to see how sensory issues may be a causal factor in any behaviour issues that arise particularly if they have not been recognised.
> Miller (2010, p31)

Although not all behaviours result from the child's sensory differences, many behaviours do appear to be caused by the child's inability to process information effectively from their senses.

Taking a problem-solving approach and considering if a sensory difference is causing an issue can lead to a better understanding of the child's behaviour.

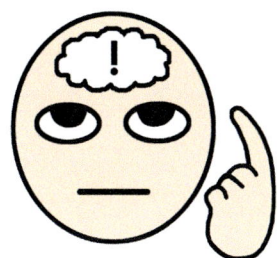

Think autism, think sensory

The next chapter explains how to complete the Sensory Questionnaire, which helps to identify concerns and identify behaviour that may be a barrier to learning or significantly affect functioning in everyday life.

References

Bogdashina, O. (2005), *Sensory Perceptual Issues in Autism and Asperger syndrome: Different Sensory Experiences, Different Perceptual Worlds*, London: Jessica Kingsley Publishers.

Bogdashina, O. (2016), *Sensory Perceptual Issues in Autism and Asperger Syndrome: Different Sensory Experiences*, 2nd edition, London: Jessica Kingsley Publishers.

Boucher, J. (2017), *Autism Spectrum Disorder*, London: Sage.

Brewer, R., Cook, R., and Bird, G. (2016), Alexithymia: A General Deficit of Interoception, *Royal Society Open Science* 3: 150664.

Grandin, T., (2006), *Thinking in Pictures*, 2nd edition, London: Bloomsbury Publishing.

Green, D., Chandler, S., Charman, T., Simonofff, E., and Baird, G. (2016), *Brief Report: DSM-5 Sensory Behaviours in Children With and Without an Autism Spectrum Disorder*, New York: Published online: 30 July 2016
Ó Springer Science+Business Media.

Fiene, L., and Brownlow, C. (2015), Investigating Interoception and Body Awareness in Adults With and Without Autism Spectrum Disorder, *Research in Autism* 8(6).

Fletcher-Watson, S., and Happé, F. (2019), *Autism: A New Introduction to Psychological Theory and Current Debate*, Abingdon: Routledge.

Frith, U. (1989), *Autism: Explaining the Enigma*, London: Blackwell.

Gardner, N. (2007), *A Friend Like Henry*, London: Hodder & Stoughton.

Godwin Emmons, P., and McKendry Anderson, L. (2005), *Understanding Learning Development and Sensory Dysfunction in Autism Spectrum Disorders, ADHD, Learning Disabilities and Bipolar Disorder*, London: Jessica Kingsley Publishers.

Grandin, T. (1996), *Thinking in Pictures*, New York: Vintage Books.

Isaacs, P. (2015), in Attwood, T., Evans, C. R., and Lesko., A. (Eds.), *Aspie's Guide to Living with Sensory Issues*, London: Jessica Kingsley Publishers.

Larkey, S. (2007), *Practical Sensory Programmes for Students with Autistic Spectrum Disorder and Other Special Needs*, London: Jessica Kingsley Publishers.

Lawrence, C. (2019), *Teacher Education and Autism: A Research Based Practical Handbook*, London: Jessica Kingsley Publishers.

Lawson, W. (2000), *Life Behind Glass*, London: Jessica Kingsley Publishers.

Lawson, W. (2001), *Understanding and Working with the Spectrum of Autism*, London: Jessica Kingsley Publishers.

Longhorn, F. (2000), Multisensory Education and Learners with Profound Autism, in Powell, A., and Jordan, R. (Eds.), *Autism and Learning: A Guide to Good Practice*, London: David Fulton Publishers.

Mahler, K. (2018), *Interview*, Middletown Centre for Autism: Sensory Processing Volume 2 Research Bulletin 26.

Miller, L. (2010), *Practical Behaviour Management Solutions for Children and Teens with Autism*, London: Jessica Kingsley Publishers.

Murphy, J., and Bird, G. (2018, July), Is Alexithymia Characterised by Impaired Interoception? Further Evidence, the Importance of Control Variables, and the Problems with the Heartbeat Counting, *Biological Psychology* 136: 189–197.

Scott, F. (2006), No Looking Back, in Ariel, C., and Naseef, R., (Eds.), *Voices from the Spectrum*, London: Jessica Kingsley Publishers.

Smith Myles, B., Cook, K., Miller, N., Rinner, L., and Robbin, L. (2000), *Asperger Syndrome and Sensory Issues: Practical Solutions for Making Sense of the World*, Kansas: Autism Asperger Publishing Co.

Thye, M., Haley, M., Bednarz, H., Herringshaw, A., Sartin, E., and Kana, R. (2018), The Impact of Atypical Sensory Processing on Social Impairments in Autism Spectrum Disorder, *Developmental Cognitive Neuroscience* 29: 151–167.

Wilkes, K. (2005), *The Sensory World of the Autistic Spectrum: A Greater Understanding*, London: The National Autistic Society.

Wiley, L. (2005) *Pretending to be Normal; Living with Asperger's Syndrome*, London: Jessica Kingsley Publishers.

3 | Creating a sensory profile of the child

The questions in the Sensory Questionnaire were designed to find out the child's response to sensory stimuli. Questions are asked to gauge the child's responses to each sensory area and help identify behaviours that suggest adaptations to the environment would be helpful. Not all of the questions will necessarily relate to a sensory area that is causing you concern, but were also designed to help you establish areas of strength or activities that the child might enjoy and therefore could be used as calming activities or as motivators.

We all have sensory preferences and dislikes, but it is important to identify those that significantly impact on the child's life. As stated previously, it is the *severity* of the response to a stimulus that determines whether the child's reaction is a problem or not and whether this impacts on the child's ability to access the learning environment and on their behaviour. For example, many young children may dislike wearing certain clothes but for children who are hypersensitive to texture, wearing of certain items could cause pain and therefore result in an extreme reaction.

Parents' and carers' input into the Sensory Questionnaire is invaluable; however, the questionnaire should also be completed by any adult who is working with the child. Sharing the questionnaire and discussing the results of the questionnaire with all adults caring and working with the child will raise awareness of the child's current reaction to experiences and enable you to identify both the child's sensory preferences and areas that impact most on their learning. Autistic children often react differently in different environments, so comparing the results from the Sensory Questionnaires that have been completed by people who see the child in different settings can help to pinpoint sensory factors that may be impacting on the child.

Completing the Sensory Questionnaire

The Sensory Questionnaire can be photocopied and completed as a paper copy.

This chapter also explains how to complete the online version of the questionnaire. The questionnaire can help you establish if the described behaviour is causing concern, the extent of the problem and how much it impacts on the child's ability to function and learn.

Parents could also use the completed questionnaire to share information with their child's educational setting or health practitioner.

Scoring the Sensory Questionnaire

The questionnaire asks you to rank the severity of the behaviour described, with **0** being not seen and **10** being the most severe. Please use either a different colour or cross to indicate the score.

0 1 2 3 4 5 6 ● 8 9 10

0 1 2 3 4 5 6 ✗ 8 9 10

Score 0 if the behaviour described is not seen

Score between 1–4 if the behaviour described is rarely seen and is having little impact on your child's learning or daily life

S**core 5** if the behaviour is seen about once a month or is a possible barrier to learning

Score between 6–9 if the behaviour described occurs more frequently and is a barrier to learning or significantly affects daily living

Score 10 if the behaviour is seen throughout the day

Please tick the right-hand box if a behaviour that is currently not causing concern was a problem in the past. This is important, as the child may revert to previously displayed behaviour if they are stressed or cannot, for some reason, use the strategy that they usually employ to cope with the situation.

Sensory Questionnaire

CHILD'S NAME: **DATE:**

Please rate by marking **0–10** the frequency the behaviour is seen **0** = behaviour not seen, **5** = seen once a month, **10** = seen throughout the day In the right-hand box, tick if the behaviour was a problem in the past.		
TOUCH	☺	☹
Hyperreactivity		
Light touch is painful, violently reacts to gentle touch	0 1 2 3 4 5 6 7 8 9 10	☐
Dislikes anything on hands and feet	0 1 2 3 4 5 6 7 8 9 10	☐
Does not like touching a range of textures	0 1 2 3 4 5 6 7 8 9 10	☐
Avoids putting hands into messy substances	0 1 2 3 4 5 6 7 8 9 10	☐
Does not like wearing certain textures of clothes, irritated by labels in clothes	0 1 2 3 4 5 6 7 8 9 10	☐
Hyporeactivity		
Decreased awareness of pain – underreacts to bruises, cuts	0 1 2 3 4 5 6 7 8 9 10	☐
Has a delayed response to textures or touch	0 1 2 3 4 5 6 7 8 9 10	☐
Unusual interests in tactile sensory aspects of the environment		
Craves tactile stimulation	0 1 2 3 4 5 6 7 8 9 10	☐
Self-injury – e.g. may hit head	0 1 2 3 4 5 6 7 8 9 10	☐
Seeks very firm hugs	0 1 2 3 4 5 6 7 8 9 10	☐
Frequently touching objects – may have routine for touching items in room	0 1 2 3 4 5 6 7 8 9 10	☐
Fascinated by certain textures	0 1 2 3 4 5 6 7 8 9 10	☐
Please describe the behaviour that is causing the greatest difficulty		

VISION	🙂	🙁
Hyperreactivity		
Does not like particular colours	0 1 2 3 4 5 6 7 8 9 10	☐
Avoids direct eye contact	0 1 2 3 4 5 6 7 8 9 10	☐
Uses peripheral vision – looks at things out of the corner of the eye	0 1 2 3 4 5 6 7 8 9 10	☐
Hits, rubs eyes when distressed	0 1 2 3 4 5 6 7 8 9 10	☐
Overly sensitive to bright lights	0 1 2 3 4 5 6 7 8 9 10	☐
Hyporeactivity		
Appears unaware of contrasting colours	0 1 2 3 4 5 6 7 8 9 10	☐
Appears not to notice obstacles	0 1 2 3 4 5 6 7 8 9 10	☐
Unusual interests in visual sensory aspects of the environment		
Looks intently at people and objects	0 1 2 3 4 5 6 7 8 9 10	☐
Moves head very close to objects to look at them	0 1 2 3 4 5 6 7 8 9 10	☐
Moves fingers in front of eyes to increase stimulation	0 1 2 3 4 5 6 7 8 9 10	☐
Fascinated with reflections	0 1 2 3 4 5 6 7 8 9 10	☐
Fascinated with brightly coloured objects, moving patterns and colours	0 1 2 3 4 5 6 7 8 9 10	☐
Please describe the behaviour that is causing the greatest difficulty		

AUITORY	🙂 😟
Hyperreactivity	
Able to hear sounds in the distance that others cannot hear	0 1 2 3 4 5 6 7 8 9 10 ☐
Covers ears to block out sounds	0 1 2 3 4 5 6 7 8 9 10 ☐
Screams in response to a particular sound	0 1 2 3 4 5 6 7 8 9 10 ☐
Makes repetitive noises to block out sounds	0 1 2 3 4 5 6 7 8 9 10 ☐
Dislikes noisy places	0 1 2 3 4 5 6 7 8 9 10 ☐
Hyporeactivity	
Does not acknowledge certain sounds	0 1 2 3 4 5 6 7 8 9 10 ☐
Has a delayed response to a sound, verbal information or instruction	0 1 2 3 4 5 6 7 8 9 10 ☐
Unusual interests in auditory sensory aspects of the environment	
Likes sounds to be repeated – bangs doors or objects continually, turns TV on and off, replays TV clips	0 1 2 3 4 5 6 7 8 9 10 ☐
Puts ear close to a sound to listen	0 1 2 3 4 5 6 7 8 9 10 ☐
Enjoys loud noises	0 1 2 3 4 5 6 7 8 9 10 ☐
Frequently makes repetitive noises; e.g. humming, clicking sounds, chants favourite words	0 1 2 3 4 5 6 7 8 9 10 ☐
Fascinated with certain sounds	0 1 2 3 4 5 6 7 8 9 10 ☐
Please describe the behaviour that is causing the greatest difficulty	

TASTE	😊	☹
Hyperreactivity		
Restricted diet	0 1 2 3 4 5 6 7 8 9 10 ☐	
Gags when eating certain foods	0 1 2 3 4 5 6 7 8 9 10 ☐	
Certain textures cause discomfort	0 1 2 3 4 5 6 7 8 9 10 ☐	
Does not like trying new foods, e.g. crunchy foods	0 1 2 3 4 5 6 7 8 9 10 ☐	
Shows extreme reaction when cleaning teeth	0 1 2 3 4 5 6 7 8 9 10 ☐	
Hyporeactivity		
Eats any food presented to them	0 1 2 3 4 5 6 7 8 9 10 ☐	
Shows no preference for particular tastes	0 1 2 3 4 5 6 7 8 9 10 ☐	
Unusual interests in gustatory sensory aspects of the environment		
Craves certain foods	0 1 2 3 4 5 6 7 8 9 10 ☐	
Licks objects/people	0 1 2 3 4 5 6 7 8 9 10 ☐	
Likes chewing on things for a long time	0 1 2 3 4 5 6 7 8 9 10 ☐	
Chews non-edible objects	0 1 2 3 4 5 6 7 8 9 10 ☐	
Fascinated with certain foods	0 1 2 3 4 5 6 7 8 9 10 ☐	
Please describe the behaviour that is causing the greatest difficulty		

SMELL	☺	☹
Hyperreactivity		
Smells are intensified and become overpowering	0 1 2 3 4 5 6 7 8 9 10 ☐	
Strong dislike for certain smells which we may think of as pleasant	0 1 2 3 4 5 6 7 8 9 10 ☐	
Certain smells cause the child to feel nauseous	0 1 2 3 4 5 6 7 8 9 10 ☐	
Hits nose when distressed	0 1 2 3 4 5 6 7 8 9 10 ☐	
Gags when smelling certain smells	0 1 2 3 4 5 6 7 8 9 10 ☐	
Hyporeactivity		
Does not notice extreme odours	0 1 2 3 4 5 6 7 8 9 10 ☐	
Has difficulty recognising food smells	0 1 2 3 4 5 6 7 8 9 10 ☐	
Unusual interests in olfactory sensory aspects of the environment		
Needs to smell themselves and others	0 1 2 3 4 5 6 7 8 9 10 ☐	
Frequently smells objects	0 1 2 3 4 5 6 7 8 9 10 ☐	
Seeks strong odours	0 1 2 3 4 5 6 7 8 9 10 ☐	
Smells and plays with faeces	0 1 2 3 4 5 6 7 8 9 10 ☐	
Fascinated by certain smells	0 1 2 3 4 5 6 7 8 9 10 ☐	
Please describe the behaviour that is causing the greatest difficulty		

VESTIBULAR	☺	☹
Hyperreactivity		
May be frightened of activities where their feet leave the ground	0 1 2 3 4 5 6 7 8 9 10	☐
Avoids balancing activities	0 1 2 3 4 5 6 7 8 9 10	☐
Dislikes swinging activities	0 1 2 3 4 5 6 7 8 9 10	☐
Dislikes activities involving changes in head position	0 1 2 3 4 5 6 7 8 9 10	☐
Has difficulty walking on uneven surfaces	0 1 2 3 4 5 6 7 8 9 10	☐
Hyporeactivity		
Does not get dizzy if spins for extended amount of time	0 1 2 3 4 5 6 7 8 9 10	☐
Appears unaware of risks when climbing, running	0 1 2 3 4 5 6 7 8 9 10	☐
Unusual interests in vestibular sensory aspects of the environment		
Craves rocking or spinning sensations	0 1 2 3 4 5 6 7 8 9 10	☐
Frequently turns upside down	0 1 2 3 4 5 6 7 8 9 10	☐
Paces up and down	0 1 2 3 4 5 6 7 8 9 10	☐
Unable to sit still, constantly moving	0 1 2 3 4 5 6 7 8 9 10	☐
Craves fast movement – always running rather than walking	0 1 2 3 4 5 6 7 8 9 10	☐
Please describe the behaviour that is causing the greatest difficulty		

PROPRIOCEPTIVE	☺ ☹
Hyperreactivity	
Dislikes certain movements	0 1 2 3 4 5 6 7 8 9 10 ☐
Difficulty with fine motor skills	0 1 2 3 4 5 6 7 8 9 10 ☐
Dislikes fast-moving activities	0 1 2 3 4 5 6 7 8 9 10 ☐
Child moves whole body to look at something	0 1 2 3 4 5 6 7 8 9 10 ☐
Dislikes rough and tumble play	0 1 2 3 4 5 6 7 8 9 10 ☐
Hyporeactivity	
Has difficulty knowing where their body is in space – unaware of position of objects and other people	0 1 2 3 4 5 6 7 8 9 10 ☐
Unaware of how much force to use when doing a task, e.g. holds pencil too tightly	0 1 2 3 4 5 6 7 8 9 10 ☐
Unusual interests in proprioceptive sensory aspects of the environment	
Likes to be hugged very tightly or squeezed	0 1 2 3 4 5 6 7 8 9 10 ☐
Seeks rough and tumble play	0 1 2 3 4 5 6 7 8 9 10 ☐
Likes to get into small, tight spaces	0 1 2 3 4 5 6 7 8 9 10 ☐
Likes to lean on furniture/against walls	0 1 2 3 4 5 6 7 8 9 10 ☐
Fascinated by movement	0 1 2 3 4 5 6 7 8 9 10 ☐
Please describe the behaviour that is causing the greatest difficulty	

INTEROCEPTION	☺	☹
Hyperreactivity		
May feel pain more acutely or for longer periods of time than other people	0 1 2 3 4 5 6 7 8 9 10 ☐	
May be excessively bothered by a small injury	0 1 2 3 4 5 6 7 8 9 10 ☐	
May feel hot or cold more intensely than others	0 1 2 3 4 5 6 7 8 9 10 ☐	
Does not like the sensation of being hungry and may eat excessively to avoid the sensation	0 1 2 3 4 5 6 7 8 9 10 ☐	
Does not like the sensation of being thirsty and may drink excessively to avoid the sensation	0 1 2 3 4 5 6 7 8 9 10 ☐	
Hyporeactivity		
May not be aware of pain signals unless they are extremely intense	0 1 2 3 4 5 6 7 8 9 10 ☐	
May not recognise they are hungry or thirsty, too hot or too cold	0 1 2 3 4 5 6 7 8 9 10 ☐	
May not recognise they are ill	0 1 2 3 4 5 6 7 8 9 10 ☐	
May be aware that something is wrong but be unable to accurately identify where these sensory signals are coming from	0 1 2 3 4 5 6 7 8 9 10 ☐	
Unusual interests in interoceptive sensory aspects of the environment		
May eat excessively	0 1 2 3 4 5 6 7 8 9 10 ☐	
May drink excessively	0 1 2 3 4 5 6 7 8 9 10 ☐	
Fascinated by internal bodily sensations	0 1 2 3 4 5 6 7 8 9 10 ☐	
Please describe the behaviour that is causing the greatest difficulty		

Instructions for completing the online Sensory Questionnaire

Access the Companion Website by visiting www.routledge.com/cw/speechmark and selecting *Autism Through a Sensory Lens*

Request access or log in using your password

Select Sensory Questionnaire

To select a score from 0–10 for each of the questions, move the slider with your curser to the required score

Use the box on the right-hand side to indicate whether the behaviour that is not currently causing a concern was a problem in the past

At the bottom of the page, you will have the opportunity to enter notes to describe the behaviour; click in the box and type in your notes, then click Next to continue

Proceed through all screens until the assessment is complete

Click the Download button to download the completed questionnaire

To create a visual representation of the questionnaire results:

Download the file Visual Representation Charts

Referring back to the Sensory Questionnaire, use the 0–10 scale on the right-hand side to shade the appropriate number of boxes relevant to each category; this can either be done on the computer or by printing the document and shading by hand

Letter explaining how to complete the Sensory Questionnaire (see Resource 7.1: letter explaining how to complete the questionnaire on p 72):
The letter included in the book is intended for educational settings to send to parents or carers. Alternatively, you can personalise and download the letter online to send to other adults that support the child explaining how to fill in the Sensory Questionnaire.

Additional information that can feed into a profile of the child

Information from occupational therapy reports
It is important to refer a child to an occupational therapist if you are concerned about the child's sensory difficulties. Some children may have already been referred to an occupational therapist, and their advice should be incorporated into the child's profile.

Observations of the child (see Resource 7.2: sensory observation form p 73 to download and print)
Observations are particularly valuable, as young autistic children are often unable to explain why they behave as they do and do not realise that they have a different way of perceiving sensory experiences than others. The information gained from your observations of the child could help you see the world from an autistic child's point of view and enable you to identify sensory preferences and plan activities that are enjoyable or calming. It could also help you to identify environmental changes that are needed.

Information from other assessments that allow you to gain a complete picture of the child

This could include play skills, speech and language therapy assessments, social skills, fine and gross motor skills assessments.

Information on the child's strengths and interests (see Resource 7.3: child's strengths and interests on p 74 for print version or complete online)

It is so important to think about 'what the child can do', as so often it is only the behaviour that challenges that people focus on and this can mask how the child is perceived and their strengths are not recognised. Ideally, discuss with the child what they think are their strengths and interests.

Information from the child's sensory preferences and dislikes (see Resource 7.4: sensory preferences and dislikes on p 75 for print version or complete online)

Use the information gained from the child's strengths and interests assessment to make a list of sensory activities which may motivate or calm the child.

* * *

In the next chapter, we will look at how you can interpret the visual representation that can be created from the information provided on the child's Sensory Questionnaire.

Creating a visual representation of the results makes it easier for you to analyse whether the child is hyperreactive or hyporeactive, and if they display unusual interests in sensory aspects of the environment. By analysing the elements in which the child has a high score, you can prioritise areas which may impact on the child's ability to cope with situations and enable you to put in place adaptations and supportive strategies.

4 | Understanding the needs of the individual child

Completing the Sensory Questionnaire can help you clearly identify concerns and behaviour that may be a barrier to learning or significantly affect the child's day-to-day functioning. Consider each sensory area and identify in what areas the child has a high score. (See Resource 7.12: blank visual representations p 98.)

Transfer the information from the Sensory Questionnaire to create a visual representation for each of the sensory areas. Use a black pen to colour in the child's scores.

For example, if the child scored 10 for the statement 'Frightened of activities where feet leave the ground' in the Sensory Questionnaire, colour in the middle column up to the 10.

10	
9	
8	
7	
6	
5	
4	
3	
2	
1	
0	
	Frightened of activities where feet leave the ground

When you have transferred the child's sensory questionnaire results to the visual representation, you will be able to see what colour section the behaviour falls into on the visual representation if the behaviour scored the following:

Scored 0 indicating the behaviour described is not seen – it will be in the blue section

Scored 1–4 indicating the behaviour described is rarely seen and is having little impact on your child's learning or daily life – it will be in the green section

Scored 5 indicating the behaviour is seen about once a month or is a possible barrier to learning – it will be in the yellow section

Scored between 6–9 indicating the behaviour described occurs more frequently and is a barrier to learning or significantly affects daily living – it will be in the orange section

Scored 10 indicating the behaviour is seen throughout the day – it will be in the red section

The following illustrates an example of the Touch section of the questionnaire for child A and the visual representation.

Example of the touch element of the Sensory Questionnaire

SENSORY QUESTIONNAIRE

CHILD'S NAME: Child A   **DATE:** Jan 2020

Please rate by marking 0-10 the frequency the behaviour is seen.
0= behaviour not seen 5=seen once a month 10= seen throughout the day
In the right hand box tick if the behaviour was a problem in the past

TOUCH	☺	☹	TICK IF A PROBLEM IN THE PAST
Hyperreactivity			
Light touch is painful, violently reacts to gentle touch	● 1 2 3 4 5 6 7 8 9 10		☐
Dislikes anything on hands and feet	● 1 2 3 4 5 6 7 8 9 10		☐
Does not like touching a range of textures	● 1 2 3 4 5 6 7 8 9 10		☐
Avoids putting hands into messy substances	● 1 2 3 4 5 6 7 8 9 10		☐
Does not like wearing certain textures of clothes, irritated by labels in clothes	● 1 2 3 4 5 6 7 8 9 10		☐
Hyporeactivity			
Decreased awareness of pain- under reacts to bruises, cuts	0 1 2 3 4 5 6 7 8 ●10		☐
Has a delayed response to textures or touch	0 1 2 3 4 ● 6 7 8 9 10		☐
Unusual interests in tactile sensory aspects of the environment			
Craves tactile stimulation	0 1 2 3 4 5 6 7 8 9 ●		☐
Self-injury – e.g. may hit head	● 1 2 3 4 5 6 7 8 9 10		☐
Seeks very firm hugs	0 1 2 3 4 5 6 7 8 9 ●		☐
Frequently touching objects – may have routine for touching items in room	0 1 2 3 4 5 6 7 ● 9 10		☐
Fascinated by certain textures	0 1 2 3 4 5 6 7 ● 9 10		☐

Example of how the visual representation illustrates the sensory profile of child A

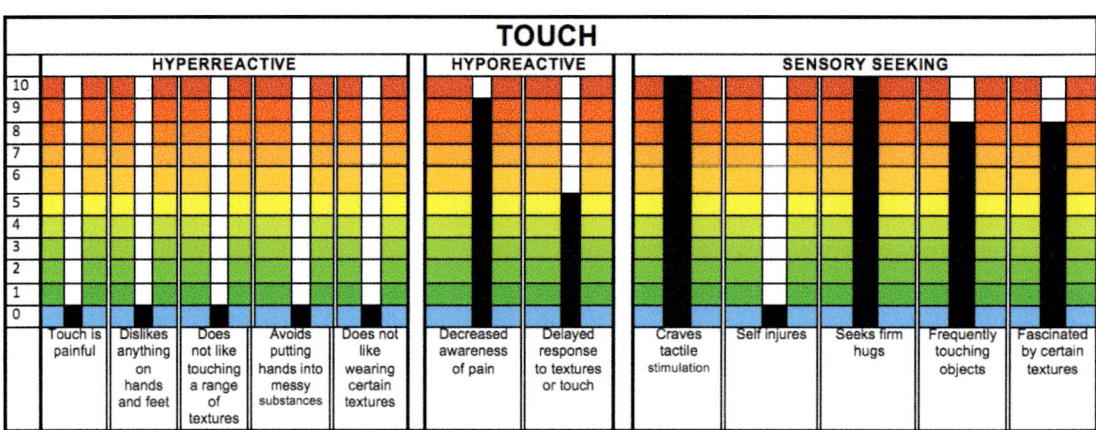

The questionnaire results can help you to identify areas where the child may need support or sensory areas that may be used for motivators or for calming activities. In the example illustrated, the child scores highly and is coloured red on the hyporeactive criteria. We can also see that the results for child A indicate they are seeking extra sensory stimulation to make sense of their environment. Ways to create a supportive environment for the child who is hyporeactive are described in Chapter 5, and lots of fun activities for the sensory-seeking child are described in Chapter 7.

Example of how the visual representation illustrates the sensory profile of child B
In this example looking at the Auditory results for child B, it clearly shows hyperreactivity to sound and that the child would benefit from changes to the environment and strategies to help with her hypersensitivity. Child B particularly found unpredictable sounds such a dog barking or hand dryers starting distressing, and this had an impact on her ability to explore the environment. In Chapter 6, there are suggested adaptations and strategies to support the hyperreactive child.

AUDITORY	☺　　　　　　　　　☹	TICK IF A PROBLEM IN THE PAST
Hyperreactivity		
Able to hear sounds that others cannot hear	0 1 2 3 4 5 6 7 8 9 ●	☐
Covers ears to block out sounds	0 1 2 3 4 5 6 7 8 9 ●	☐
Screams in response to a particular sound	0 1 2 3 4 5 6 7 8 9 ●	☐
Makes repetitive noises to block out sounds	0 1 2 3 4 5 ● 7 8 9 10	☐
Dislikes noisy places	0 1 2 3 4 5 6 7 8 9 ●	☐
Hyporeactivity		
Does not acknowledge certain sounds	● 1 2 3 4 5 6 7 8 9 10	☐
Has a delayed response to a sound, verbal information or instruction	● 1 2 3 4 5 6 7 8 9 10	☐
Unusual interests in tactile sensory aspects of the environment		
Likes sounds to be repeated – bangs doors or objects continually, turns TV on and off, replays TV clips	● 1 2 3 4 5 6 7 8 9 10	☐
Puts ear close to a sound to listen	● 1 2 3 4 5 6 7 8 9 10	☐
Enjoys loud noises	● 1 2 3 4 5 6 7 8 9 10	☐
Frequently makes repetitive noises; e.g. humming, clicking sounds, chants favourite words	0 1 2 3 4 5 ● 7 8 9 10	☐
Fascinated with certain sounds	● 1 2 3 4 5 6 7 8 9 10	☐

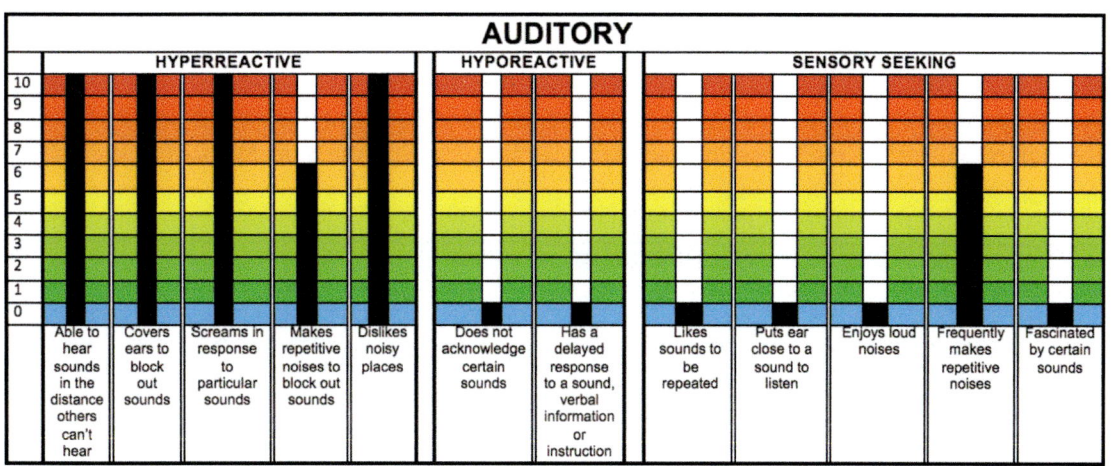

Occupational therapy

If the child scores within the orange and red bands, it indicates that the child is experiencing significant differences in their sensory input – and I hope that this book will increase your understanding and give some helpful strategies to help the child cope in day-to-day situations. If you are concerned about the child's development, refer to an occupational therapist. Children can be referred to occupational therapy by a range of people such as paediatricians, general practitioners, health visitors, school staff and speech and language therapists.

An occupational therapist works on areas such as fine and gross motor skills, motor planning, self-regulation and sensory processing. The occupational therapist will also identify any barriers that prevent the child from participating in day-to-day activities.

The occupational therapist will assess the child and evaluate what type of therapy would be appropriate.

Occupational therapists often assess using Dunn's 'Sensory Profile'. The assessment measures a child's sensory processing ability and its effect on how the child functions in daily life. The questionnaire describes the child's responses to various sensory experiences. Scores compare the autistic child's performance to the typically developing child. Tomchek and Dunn (2007) reported results showing that on 92% of the items in the profile the autistic children performed 'significantly differently' Tomchek and Dunn (2007, p198) than did children without disabilities. Dunn designed the profile in order to provide insights into a child's performance and provide information to enable practitioners to plan a more effective intervention programme.

The occupational therapist may believe that the child would benefit from sensory integration therapy. An intervention such as sensory integration therapy is described by Wilkes as involving

> gentle exposure to various sensory stimuli. The aim of this therapy is to strengthen, balance and develop the central nervous system's processing of sensory stimuli.
> Wilkes (2005, p6)

The occupational therapist will design a routine of activities for the child. Using techniques to calm a child or conversely stimulate the child's senses within a planned programme is often called a 'sensory diet'. The activities in a sensory diet can help children who are hyperreactive to feel calmer, and children who are hyporeactive feel more alert, so that they are in an optimal state to concentrate and learn.

The occupational therapist can also offer advice and information to educational settings to develop the staff's knowledge and suggest ways they can support the child within their environment.

Larkey (2007) believes that sensory programmes are important because they

> encourage children to have interactions with their environment, acknowledge fears and slowly work on reducing them, often provide long term changes.
> Larkey (2007, p12)

Conversely, Lawrence (2019) argues that

> We need to accept and nurture the sensory differences of our autistic pupils, rather than focusing on desensitisation. Their sensitivities may be difficult for them to manage as children but may be nurtured into outstanding skills as adults.
> Lawrence (2019, p19)

There is a debate over the advocacy of sensory integration therapy and whether it can help children with sensory processing issues as research findings differ. A systematic review of research studies conducted by Lang et al. (2012) concluded that sensory integration therapy did not result in a consistent positive effect as a treatment for autistic children. Continued studies are needed to further investigate the effectiveness of sensory interventions.

Attwood (2015) points out that for an autistic person,

> repeated experience of an aversive experience (desensitization) does not lead to habituation, and if an experience is particularly unpleasant, it is almost impossible to ignore. You need compassion and cooperation to help you either avoid or tolerate sensory experiences. Attwood (2015, p36)

The next chapter will consider ways that you can create a sensory-supportive environment, and suggests strategies to support the hyperreactive child who has an adverse reaction to sensory stimuli or the child who is hyporeactive.

References

Attwood, T., Evans, C. R., and Lesko., A. (Eds.) *Aspie's Guide to Living with Sensory Issues*, London: Jessica Kingsley Publishers.

Lang, R., O'Reilly, M., Healy, O., Rispoli, M., Lydon, H., Streusand, W., Davis, T., Kang, S., Sigafoos, J., Lancioni, G., Didden, R., and Giesbers, S. (2012), Sensory Integration Therapy for Autism Spectrum Disorders: A Systematic Review, *Research in Autism Spectrum Disorders* 6: 1004–1018.

Larkey, S. (2007), *Practical Sensory Programmes for Students with Autistic Spectrum Disorder and Other Special Needs*, London: Jessica Kingsley Publishers.

Lawrence, C., (2019), *Teacher Education and Autism: A Research-Based Practical Handbook*, London: Jessica Kingsley Publishers.

Tomchek, S. D., and Dunn, W. (2007), Sensory Processing in Children With and Without Autism: A Comparative Study Using the Short Sensory Profile, *American Journal of Occupational Therapy* 61: 190–200.

Wilkes, K. (2005), *The Sensory World of the Autistic Spectrum: A Greater Understanding*, London: The National Autistic Society.

5 | Creating a sensory-supportive environment

As Lawson (2008) explains, it is the result of interactions with an environment that exacerbates autistic difficulties and that

> as an autistic individual I am disabled due to the non accommodation of my difficulties.
> Lawson (2008, p62)

For many autistic children, sensory sensitivities can have a huge impact on their ability to cope. They may not have developed the skills to communicate their discomfort to others or found strategies to help to minimise the sensory experiences they find unpleasant. It is only by observing the child's behaviour through a sensory lens that we can help to identify their challenges and offer appropriate support to the child. Wood (2019) describes the sensory sensitivities that the child may encounter in their educational setting:

> the school environment can present autistic children with a multi-sensory onslaught in terms of sounds, smells, textures and visual impacts that constitutes both a distraction and a source of discomfort.
> Wood (2019, p46)

Honeybourne (2018) explains what impact these sensory sensitivities can have:

> The environment around us can have a considerable impact on our wellbeing, as well as on our ability to learn and concentrate.
> Honeybourne (2018, p83)

In this chapter, we will consider how we can put in place simple changes to create a sensory-supportive environment for the individual and strategies to support the hyperreactive and hyporeactive child. The importance of providing an enabling environment is stated in the statutory framework for the Early Years Foundation Stage where it says:

> Children learn and develop well in enabling environments, in which their experiences respond to their individual needs and there is a strong partnership between practitioners and parents and/or carers.
> (Department of Education 2017, p6)

Analysing the child's sensory profile that you have created can help you to work out how to support the child. If the results of the child's Sensory Questionnaire indicate that the child has a significant difficulty with sensory reactivity by implementing some of the ideas suggested in this chapter, it could make an enormous difference to their everyday lives. Look at the environment through a sensory lens and think about what changes could be made to create a sensory-friendly environment. Every child's sensory needs are unique, and as Miller (2010) points out:

> The implications sensory issues may have in relation to behaviour are significant, and understanding an individual's sensory profile is an important element when planning an appropriate environment.
> Miller (2010, p31)

Ideas to support the child who is oversensitive and hyperreactive

Touch

- Some autistic children may avoid messy activities or activities that involve touching particular textures. If the child is nervous about approaching an activity, demonstrate it and allow plenty of time for them to observe the activity.

- Find ways to adapt the activity so that they can still do the learning without having to experience something they are uncomfortable with; e.g. the child could wear gloves while exploring play dough or use objects to touch it rather than their fingers.

- Remember the child may be very sensitive to light touch. Give the child a warning if you are going to touch them. In the classroom, problems can often arise when the children have to line up and others might brush against the autistic child. Perhaps the child could either be at the end or the beginning of the line or not be part of the line and leave the classroom before or after the other children.

- Certain textures of clothing may be uncomfortable. Allow the child to wear fabrics they like – when you find clothing the child likes, buy several items in different sizes as they can get very attached to a particular item of clothing.

- Autistic children are often particularly sensitive to labels and seams in clothes. Remove labels in clothing and wear socks inside out to lessen the effect of the seams.

Sight

- Creating a low-arousal environment can be really helpful. Consider using calming colours such as cream or pastel colours for walls, floors and upholstery. Avoid brightly coloured patterns, as these can be confusing.

- Use natural lighting or soft lighting if possible. Avoid fluorescent lighting, as many people find the flickering uncomfortable.

- Consider the window covering. Voile curtains can help to filter the light, or fit semi-transparent window film, which can also defuse the bright sunlight. If possible, avoid blinds with slats as they can cause distracting light patterns in bright sunlight.

- Create an organised and uncluttered environment.

- Encourage the child to wear sunglasses or glasses with tinted lenses. Wearing a hat with a large brim or a cap can also limit the amount of light reaching the eyes. Lawson describes how wearing a baseball cap was a helpful strategy:

> As a younger person I 'lived' in my baseball cap. My cap served to slightly limit my field of vision to help prevent sensory overwhelm, gave pressure to my head so I knew where I ended

and helped me navigate open space. If I was made to remove my cap, my attention went with it and I became inattentive in class.
Lawson (2019, p11)

Hearing

- Background noises such as ticking clocks, humming electrical devices, projectors and lawn mowers can be very irritating and prevent the child from concentrating. Consider how these sounds can be reduced.

- Acknowledge the child's fear. Always warn the child about when to expect a sensory stimulus they do not like. Sometimes if the child is in control of when the noise is going to happen, it can reduce anxiety. One child I knew hated it when his mum did the hoovering but could cope if he turned on the machine and then he would be able to calmly go to another room.

- Autistic children often use the strategy of covering their ears with their hands to block out sudden noises such as emergency vehicle sirens. Encourage the child to wear ear defenders or earphones to block out sounds in noisy environments. Earphones can be worn without having music playing, but many autistic people discover that playing music that they find calming can help to block out sounds they find uncomfortable.

- Consider the surfaces used in buildings. Carpets can reduce the impact of sound rather than the use of hard surfaces such as tiles and wooden flooring.

- Consider where you can provide a quiet area for the child to go to if they find the noise level in the building too loud.

- Avoid noisy environments if possible. If you need to visit a noisy place, think about when it will be at its least noisy. Always warn the autistic child that it is likely to be noisy and take calming toys or objects with you which can help to calm and distract the child from the sensory experience they are finding unpleasant. There are many organisations that are offering 'autism-friendly times' when they have reduced the sensory stimulation.

Taste

- Do not pressure a child to eat foods that they find unpalatable.

- Some children do not like different textures of food mixed together. Offer one type of food on each plate.

- Use food in sensory play activities; e.g. provide mashed potatoes for the child to explore instead of non-food materials such as play dough.

- Adapt cooking activities so that the child can participate without handling the textures they do not like.

- As Cormack (2019) explains:

> The core goal for teachers should be to foster positive and low anxiety interactions with food rather than pushing children to do things they are not comfortable with.
> Cormack (2019, p104)

Smell

- Respect the child if they say a smell that you find pleasant is intensified and unpleasant to them, and try to find a way for the child to avoid it. The smell of certain foods cooking can be distressing, and the child may need to leave the room. Putting a scent of something the child does like on to a wristband or tissue that they can smell when encountering an unpleasant smell can help to mask the unpleasant one.

- The child may find the smell of food difficult to cope with in the school dining room. Consider other areas in which they could eat their lunch.

- Use unperfumed soaps, shampoos, washing powder and cleaning products.

Vestibular

- Put support in place for children who find balancing activities difficult – offer to hold their hand to support them when they are exploring playground equipment.

- Be aware of the child's difficulty tolerating movement and balancing during physical education lessons, and do not insist they have to complete an activity they are uncomfortable with.

Proprioception

- If the child is always bumping into furniture, consider how you position items in the room to avoid obstacles.

- Provide support for writing activities – different pencil and pen grips made from soft foam or plastic can reduce the discomfort when holding them. A sloped or angled writing surface may increase comfort when working.

- If the child has the need to move all the time, it can be difficult for them to concentrate on anything else. Offer regular movement breaks to allow the child to take a few minutes to move and then refocus.

- Encourage the child to do some physical exercise before they need to concentrate on an activity. Jumping, running and skipping will all give input to the muscles and be calming for the child. Jumping on a trampoline can be particularly calming for the child.

- The deep pressure provided by weighted jackets can have a calming effect on the proprioceptive system, reducing the child's anxiety. Carrying a backpack with some books or toys in can also help. The weight offers gentle pressure which helps to soothe the child. Take care not to make the bag too heavy, as too much weight could damage joints. Putting a weighted soft toy over their knees when sitting can also help.

- Some children seek small enclosed spaces and like to squeeze themselves into tight places. Being wrapped in a blanket can reduce the child's anxiety.

- A large beanbag or cushion which the child can snuggle into can help to calm the child.

Interoception

- Use visual support for situations or tasks that the child may be oversensitive to, such as eating or drinking. If possible use the child's special interests; for example, say 'Thomas the Tank Engine needs to have some water' to encourage the child to have a drink. Use a reward to help establish motivation.

- Use Social Stories™ to explain the importance of regular eating and drinking. Social Stories™ were created by Carol Gray (2015). They are descriptions of a situation, event or activity which include information about what to expect in that situation and why. They can be very helpful as a visual focus for talking about situations that the child is finding difficult.

- Breathing techniques and exercises are helpful for calming, as well as paying attention to what is going on inside our bodies.

- Yoga, which involves holding postures that stretch muscles and limbs, doing breathing exercises and meditation, helps focus the child on listening to their body. It encourages children to relax and pay attention to the present and how their body is feeling, helping the child learn calming techniques and strategies to manage strong emotions and feelings.

- Read story books like *The Panicosaurus*, written by Kay Al-Ghani (2012), which explains anxiety to the child and suggests techniques for lessening anxiety.

- Mindfulness can be helpful and is now often taught as part of the personal, social and emotional development curriculum in schools. The exercises can help the child develop a greater awareness of what is happening here and now, rather than worrying about what has happened or what might happen. Mindfulness exercises can help the child to regulate their emotions.

Environments causing sensory overload

Chris Packham (2020) describes how stimuli from different sensory systems can cause real difficulty:

> I rarely go into supermarkets. I find that environment really challenging, all of the bright lights, the confusion of the enormous complexity of goods in there, plus all the smells and the sounds. It's a difficult environment.
> Packham (2020)

Some autistic children reach and often exceed the sensory stimulation they can cope with, resulting in sensory overload and an extreme reaction. Some environments or events are just too much for the child. Try limiting the time the child needs to be in that situation so that it is a positive experience rather than a negative one; e.g. if the child has been invited to a party and wants to go, explain to the host that they do want to come but describe the child's sensitivities and state that they may need to arrive late or leave early.

Sensory first aid

Sometimes it is impossible to avoid an environment or situation that you know will be difficult for the child to cope with and could result in their hypersensitivity causing distress.

A good motto is to be prepared.

Explain to the child what they are likely to encounter in a specific environment and in the same way as you might carry medical supplies in a first aid kit so that you can quickly respond after an accident, make up a bag or box for the child which contains items to distract and calm the child. If the child is hypersensitive to sound, items such as ear defenders or earphones and a phone to listen to music which can reduce the intensity of the stimulus. Attwood et al. (2015, p57) suggests having items that offer 'alternative sensory experiences that neutralises specific sensory sensitivity' and are 'mesmerising enough to block out sensory experiences'. Other items could be a squidgy ball to squeeze, glitter tubes to watch the rainbow glitter move, tactile fidget toys, Blu Tack, or a drink with a straw.

Maguire (2015) describes what he uses for 'sensory first aid':

> I carry ear plugs or a music player to use in the event of loud noises. I carry a calming stim object: personally, I carry a camera for this purpose – you may want something else. Carry

scents that calm you. Wear clothes that are sensory-friendly. Carry dark or coloured glasses if they help.
Maguire in Attwood et al. (2015, p19)

Discovering what helps the child to calm and self-regulate is trial and error. By observing the child, you learn more about their sensory preferences and ways you can help them cope and begin to develop their self-calming strategies. Complete Resource 7.4: sensory preferences to give you some more ideas of things to put in your bag.

A calming sensory space

Create an area the child can go to that will support their sensory needs. This could be their bedroom, a pop-up tent or even a table which you could turn into a den by covering it with a blanket. Fill it with cushions, bean bags and different textured fabrics. Include things to help calm such as favourite books, mood lights, soft toys, colouring books, comics, bubbles and sensory toys.

You may find there are sensory rooms in your local area that the child can access. Sensory rooms can provide a relaxing space where the child is surrounded by pleasant sensory experiences. They often have colour changing fibre optics, bubble tubes, tactile wall panels, ball pits, mirror balls, a sound system to produce music, mats and tunnels to explore to help the child regulate their senses.

Ideas to support the child who is undersensitive and hyporeactive

Ensure that people are aware that the child is undersensitive or hyporeactive and may not respond to a sensory stimulus, or have a delayed reaction. Safety is therefore a paramount consideration.

Safety

Many children with autism lack an awareness of their own safety and indeed have a reduced awareness of pain. As explained previously, the feeling of pain is the body's way of warning us of danger – and if this response is lacking, there could be a link between the decreased awareness of pain and the fearless behaviour described by parents and staff.

The child may have an accident and not tell you or realise that they have hurt themselves. In order to ensure the child's safety, activities need close supervision.

• Lock cupboards containing hazardous materials when not in use.

• Use electric plug covers.

• Make sure the water temperature for baths and washing is not too hot.

• Label objects such as radiators, warning that they may be hot.

• Near busy roads, the child may not be aware of the traffic. For young children who do not like holding an adult's hand, the child could wear a backpack with safety reins.

Vestibular

• Providing movement activities such as swinging, jumping and spinning will stimulate the vestibular system.

- Turning upside down or doing cartwheels and handstands can give intense vestibular input.

- Provide a 'wobble cushion' for the child to sit on. These are air-filled cushions that create a moving surface. This movement can help to alert the child and 'wake up' their vestibular sense.

Proprioception

- Activities that involve input to the muscles and joints, as well as being helpful for calming the hyperreactive child, can also help the hyporeactive child and enable them to increase their attention and level of arousal. The activities that will do this are unique to each child and it is important to observe the child and identify which ones will work for the child. Movement gives proprioceptive input but some activities that involve the whole body such as pushing or pulling, oral actions such as chewing or sucking and activities involving the hands such as squeezing or pinching actions will all give increased proprioceptive input.

- Some hyporeactive children present as lethargic. Allow movement breaks and opportunities for the child to get up and stretch.

Interoception

- For the child who does not recognise their internal body sensations such as the need to go to the toilet, needing to have a drink or to eat, you can use visual prompt cards as reminders in the house or classroom.

- Help the child to recognise and to describe how their body feels, what could be the cause and what they could do to make themselves more comfortable; for example, if their skin feels itchy and it is red, they might have an allergy to a food they have eaten or have been bitten by an insect and a solution would be to tell an adult and put some ointment on their skin; or the itchiness and redness could be caused by the texture of their clothing, in which case changing their clothes could make them feel more comfortable. See Resource 7.10: recognising how my body feels for more examples and a blank chart for the child to record their own bodily feelings, to consider different causes and solutions to help them feel more comfortable.

- The child may not be able to feel their heartbeat quicken when they have done strenuous exercise. Do activities to raise or lower heartbeat/pulse and chart these visually. This may also help them to recognise the feeling and be aware of changes to their heart rate when they are feeling scared.

- The child may not recognise when they are getting too hot or too cold. Use a thermometer to check room/outdoor temperatures and decide on a particular temperature when the child needs to remove clothing or put on warmer clothing. This avoids confusion for the child when you have unseasonable weather and the child does not understand why; for example, you need warm clothing in summer if it is a particularly cold day.

- Help the child recognise their emotions. The autistic child often has difficulty identifying not only their own feelings, but also the feelings of others. Use photographs of faces showing different feelings and talk about how the face changes when different emotions are expressed. Talk to the child about how their body reacts to each emotion.

- Label the emotions. The child may not be able to interpret the facial expression, body language or tone of voice of others. Describe how you are feeling and label what you think the child is feeling; for example, when they are playing with a favourite toy, say 'I can see you are happy'.

- Use Resource 7.9: words for emotions to help the child to describe how they are feeling and talk about situations that make them happy, sad, etc.
- Talk about how the child is feeling when they are completing the sensory activities outlined in Chapter 6, which will help to raise awareness of different body areas and the feelings associated with them.

The educational setting

The classroom or nursery can be a busy, noisy and overwhelming place for the autistic child. It is vital that practitioners have received training on autism and are able to recognise and be sensitive to the child's individual needs, as without an understanding of sensory differences, they may misinterpret the child's behaviour. As Lawrence (2019) emphasises:

> It is essential that as teachers we are sensitive to these sensory issues, rather than being distracted by responding to the behaviours-avoidant, anxious, self injurious – which the sensory overload may prompt.
> Lawrence (2019, p19)

The SEND Code of Practice (Department of Education 2015, 6.9, p93) requires schools to make 'reasonable adjustments' to prevent children being at a disadvantage. Often small changes can make an enormous difference.

As Mahler says:

> I believe one of the best solutions that we can use as professionals is to proactively provide a sensory friendly school environment. Learn about each young person and his or her unique sensory needs. Try to consider these sensory needs throughout the school day and implement modifications that will maximise sensory comfort.
> Mahler (2018, p6)

Beaney and Kershaw (2014) explain that the classroom environment can have a dramatic effect on the pupil's behaviour and ability to learn, and suggest that the autistic child (and others in the class) will benefit from the following:

- The school day will be a lot easier for the autistic child if regular routines can be established – this will help to reduce anxiety often associated with social demands. Autistic children like routine and things to be predictable, and changes can make them anxious. Warn the child about any alterations to the routine of the day or changes in staffing to reduce their anxiety.
- An organised and uncluttered classroom – classrooms can be very stimulating and too many displays can be overwhelming. Keep information around a focus area, such as the whiteboard, as clear as possible. Put displays within borders.
- Well labelled and organised equipment – equipment that is needed should be easily accessible and items that would distract should be placed out of sight.
- A designated space where the child can go to if they become sensory overloaded and need to calm down – if the classroom is very crowded, try to find a quiet area elsewhere in the school that could be used as a 'haven' for the child.
- Planning multisensory activities into the school curriculum – bringing these activities in to the weekly curriculum encourages the generalisation of skills. Outings and the creative use of outside areas give the children an opportunity to explore the environment using all their senses.

The next chapter includes ideas of fun activities for the sensory-seeking child.

References

Al-Ghani, K. (2012), *The Panicosaurus: Managing Anxiety in Children Including Those with Asperger Syndrome*, London: Jessica Kingsley Publishers.

Attwood, T., Evans, C., and Lesko, A. (Eds.) (2015), *An Aspie's Guide to Living with Sensory Issues*, London: Jessica Kingsley Publishers.

Beaney, J., and Kershaw, P. (2014), *Autism in the Primary Classroom*, London: National Autistic Society.

Cormack, J. (2019), in Lawrence, C. (Ed.), *Teacher Education and Autism*, London: Jessica Kingsley Publishers.

Department for Education (2015), *SEND Code of Practice: 0 to 25 years, Statutory Guidance*, London: DfE.

Department of Education (2017), *Statutory Framework for the Early Years Foundation Stage*, London: DFE.

Gray, C. (2015), *The New Social Story Book*, Arlington: Future Horizons.

Honeybourne, V. (2018), *The Neurodiverse Classroom: A Teacher's Guide to Individual Learning Needs and How to Meet Them*, London: Jessica Kingsley Publishers.

Lawrence, C. (2019), *Teacher Education and Autism*, London: Jessica Kingsley Publishers.

Lawson, W. (2008), *Concepts of Normality*, London: Jessica Kingsley Publishing.

Lawson, W. (2019), Foreword, in Wood, R. (Ed.), *Inclusive Education for Autistic Children: Helping Children and Young People to Learn and Flourish in the Classroom*, London: Jessica Kingsley Publishers.

Maguire, R., in Attwood, T., Evans, C., and Lesko, A. (Eds.) (2015), *An Aspie's Guide to Living with Sensory Issues*, London: Jessica Kingsley Publishers.

Mahler, K. (2018), *Interview*, Middletown Centre for Autism: Sensory Processing Volume 2 Research Bulletin 26.

Miller, L. (2010), *Practical Behaviour Management Solutions for Children and Teens with Autism*, London: Jessica Kingsley Publishers.

Packham, C., (2020), *National Autistic Society*, www.autism.org.uk; https://www.autism.org.uk/get-involved/campaign/autism-hour/real-stories/chris-packham.aspx.

Wood, R. (2019), *Inclusive Education for Autistic Children: Helping Children and Young People to Learn and Flourish in the Classroom*, London: Jessica Kingsley Publishers.

6 | Fun activities for the sensory-seeking child

Traditionally, the education of young children has recognised the importance of providing a wide range of experiences and activities to encourage children to explore using their senses. The Early Years Foundation Stage Statutory Framework (Department of Education 2017, p6) has the guiding principle that children learn and develop in enabling environments, in which their experiences respond to their individual needs. I believe that for autistic children, sensory exploration and play opportunities continue to be priorities beyond the Foundation Stage and should be included by educators in curriculum planning for older children. In the home, many children will benefit from this type of play.

The fun activities in this chapter are designed for exploration and sensory play. They are all activities that I have used with children, both in an educational setting and at home. My aspirations for the sensory work that I have undertaken with autistic children has been for them to develop an understanding of their sensory issues, find strategies to manage these difficulties and be able to cope successfully and even enjoy everyday situations that previously they found difficult. By thinking creatively, making small changes to an activity or the environment and providing opportunities for sensory play can make a huge difference.

All children are unique and their sensory needs will be very different. Some children will have sensory issues across one, several or all senses. They may be hypersensitive in one and hyposensitive in another. They may also respond differently at different times.

The activities in this chapter can be used with different aims in mind:

- **Enjoyment** – Looking at the child's Sensory Questionnaire results and their sensory preferences will help you identify in which sensory areas the child is sensory seeking and the activities described in this chapter that the child may enjoy. Some children who are hypersensitive are fascinated by a sensory stimulus or activity, and can get intense pleasure from it. An intense interest in a sensory stimulus can sometimes create a difficulty, as it means the child may spend extended time just focusing on the stimuli and withdraws from other activities. It is important therefore to achieve a balance between the child participating in activities they enjoy but not spending so much time on it that it restricts their development.

- **Calming** – Fascination with a sensory stimulus can have a calming effect. The child may use repetitive sensory behaviours to lessen overstimulation. The autistic child is often very anxious, so it is important that they find a strategy that helps to reduce their anxiety.

- **Distraction** – An activity from a preferred sense may distract the child if they are having difficulty coping with a sensory stimulus that they find uncomfortable. For example, one child was very sensitive to sound and disliked noisy environments but was fascinated by moving patterns of light and he would seek out and intensely focus on patterns made by sunlight. This enabled him to block out the discomfort when encountering a noisy environment.

- **Gaining sensory information** – Some children who are hyposensitive may crave a sensory experience in order to provide their body with more information about their environment.

- **Motivation** – For autistic children, praise may not be enough. Motivation may not be intrinsic, and they will need something tangible: an activity or an object. Many of the activities described in this chapter and in the list of the child's sensory preferences (Resource 7.4 p 75) will be motivating for the child and can be used as motivators or rewards.

The child should be encouraged to make choices and express preferences. Observe the child's responses carefully. If a child shows that they have lost interest or do not like the activity, either through speech or body language, stop. Consider if there were any factors that could be changed so that the child can enjoy the activity.

Create a choice board so the child can indicate which activity they would like to do. You can print Resource 7.6: fun sensory activities choice board (p 82) and cut out the symbols illustrating the fun activities from Resource 7.5 grid of visual symbols (p 76) to use on it.

An example of a choice board for sensory play and exploration is shown here.

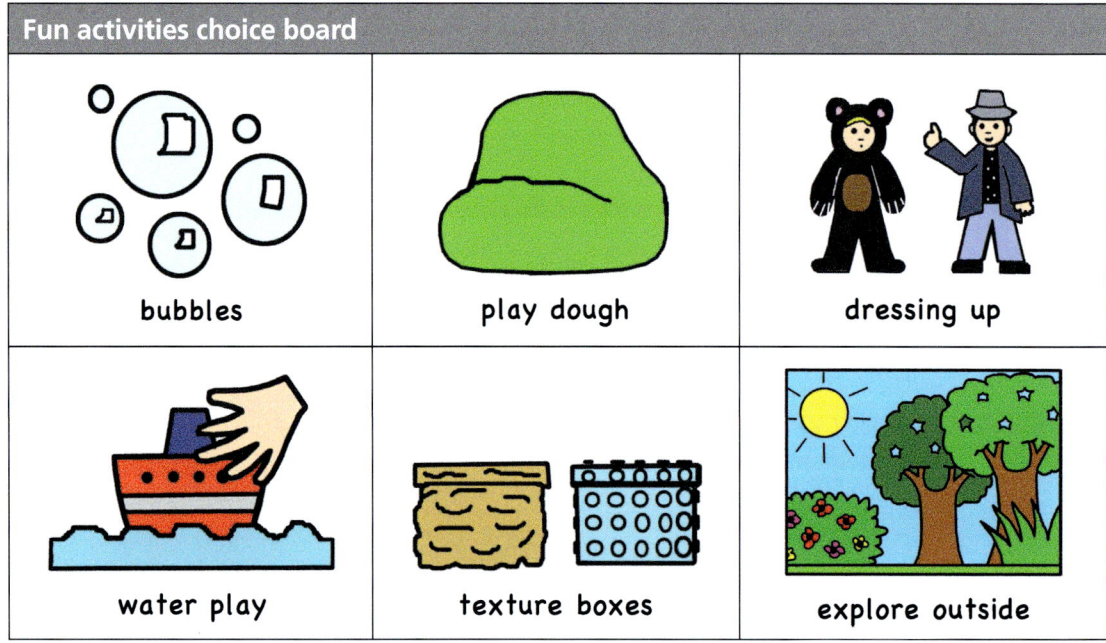

Creating boards for different situations may be helpful. The choice board can be particularly helpful if the child begins to recognise when they are getting overexcited and need to find a strategy to help them calm. This could be taken out with the child as a visual reminder of the strategies they could use and have found helpful in the past.

An example of a calming activities choice board is shown here.

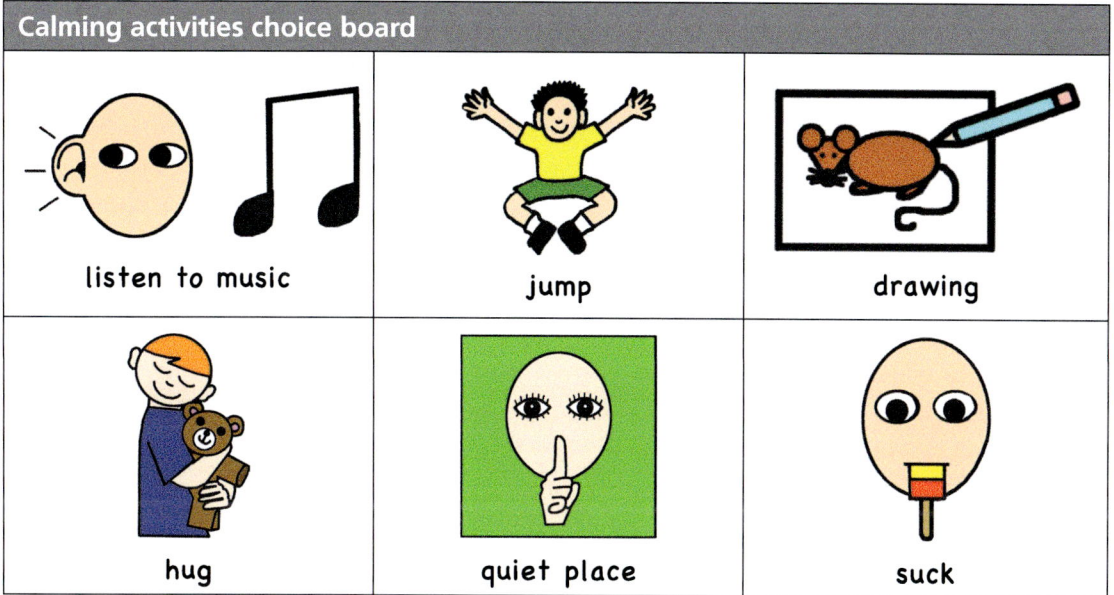

Calming activities choice board		
listen to music	jump	drawing
hug	quiet place	suck

All activities should be supervised by an adult. It is important to check if the child has any allergies or sensitivities before starting any activity.

Tactile exploration

Here are some possible observed behaviours that suggest the child would benefit from the following activities and from similar tactile exploratory activities. The child may find the activities motivating, and they can calm the child.

- Craves tactile stimulation and constantly touches people or objects
- Self-injury; for example, a child may bite themselves or bang their head on the ground
- Seeks very firm hugs
- Likes to be tightly wrapped in a blanket
- Frequently puts objects in mouth
- Fascinated by certain textures and loves to touch them

touch	SUGGESTED TACTILE ACTIVITIES
texture boxes	**Texture boxes** Explore texture boxes. Suggested contents – sand, rice, lentils, shells, pasta, jelly, oats, cornflour, water. Sometimes place contents on a large tray so child can pour substances. Introduce different utensils for handling the textures – spoons, scoops, jugs, sieves.
treasure hunt	**Treasure hunt** Make a treasure hunt. Hide objects in play dough, clay or sand for children to find.
play dough	**Play dough** Explore play dough and clay. Add textures – glitter, sand, rice, etc. Roll, squeeze, pinch, pound, poke it. Introduce different utensils for making marks – sticks, plastic knife, spoons, fork, cutters, graters.
dressing up	**Dressing up** Use a variety of textures in dressing up clothes.
feely bag	**Feely bag** Put items with different textures in the feely bag – feathers, sandpaper, felt.
texture block game	**Texture block game** Cover wood blocks with different textured fabrics. Put one set of texture blocks in a bag. Set out the matching pairs on a table. Ask the child to feel in the bag and match textures on the different blocks.
feely walk	**Feely walk** Go on a feely walk – create a route using different textures such as carpet, bubble wrap, sheepskin, etc. If the child has difficulty keeping their balance, provide close supervision.
water play	**Water play** Explore water in a tank – change colour of water, add bubbles, use different toys for pouring and exploring.
foam soap	**Foam soap** Spread foam soap over surface and draw patterns or blow it. Push cars and objects through foam. Hide objects. Make figure eights and shapes in the foam with car or object.
ball	**Texture balls** Play with balls with different textures – velcro soft and rough, sellotape sticky side out, Koosh ball.

touch	SUGGESTED TACTILE ACTIVITIES
hand tower game	**Hand towers** Play the hand tower game whereby you put one hand down, child covers it, then you put your hand on top, etc.
water painting	**Water painting** Use water and brushes to paint the playground or patio
mixing colour	**Mixing colours** Using zippy bags filled with paint is a great way to enable the child to explore without getting their hands messy. Put 2 colours in a zippy bag; seal well! The child can squidge the paint together and watch how the colours blend together.
finger painting	**Finger painting** Use fingers to paint. Use different textures of paint. If the child is not happy to put their finger in the paint, let them wear gloves or dip a pencil into the paint to make patterns.
squidgy spaghetti	**Squidgy spaghetti** Use cooked, cold spaghetti to make shapes and patterns.
light materials	**Light materials** Use light materials such as tissue paper, light scarves or silk to place on skin.
fan	**Fans** Use fans. Feel the effect of air on different parts of the body.
bubbles	**Bubbles** Blow bubbles or use a bubble machine. Catch and pop bubbles.
explore outside	**Explore outside environment** Make mud pies, feel different textures of plants, make bark rubbings.
brush	**Brushing** Let the child use the brush to stroke their skin.

Visual exploration

Here are some possible observed behaviours that suggest the child would benefit from the following activities and from similar visual exploratory activities. The child may find the activities motivating, and they can calm the child.

- Looks intently at people and objects
- Moves head very close to objects to look at them
- Moves fingers in front of eyes to increase stimulation
- Likes turning lights on and off
- Fascinated with reflections
- Fascinated with brightly coloured objects
- Fascinated with moving patterns and colours

looking	SUGGESTED VISUAL ACTIVITIES
	Have fun playing games such as 'Row, Row, Row Your Boat' and 'Pat a Cake'. Sit opposite on seesaw. Play 'Peepbo'. Attract attention to your face when playing; e.g. put objects near your face, blow bubbles close to your face, put things on your head, wear funny hats or glasses.
magnifying glass	**Magnifying glasses** Encourage careful looking.
coloured looker	**Coloured lookers** Overlap coloured lenses and tissue paper to see the effect. Look at objects using lookers. Look through fine fabrics/nets.
mirror	**Mirror games** Play games in front of a mirror so child can look at themself – wear dressing up clothes, blow bubbles, wiggle fingers, make shapes in front of the mirror.
finger rhymes	**Finger/hand rhymes** Use rhymes like 'This Little Piggy' or 'Teddy Bear, Teddy Bear'.
moving objects	**Moving objects** Watch objects that move such as mobiles, balloons, bubbles, fascination tubes, oil pictures or moving light patterns. Play 'Peepbo' with objects, jack in the box, streamers, colourful toys.
ball games	**Ball games** Play ball games – rolling skittles, throwing balls – target games.

looking	SUGGESTED VISUAL ACTIVITIES
tracking	**Tracking activities** **Side to side** – use balls, toys on string, toy cars, moving toys, torches. **Up and down** – bounce balls, bubbles, toys on springs, toys on elastic, yo-yo, play 'Incy Wincy Spider'. Play tracking games on computer programmes showing colours and patterns.
light and dark	**Light and dark** Explore light and dark. Make patterns with torch light. Use coloured lights. Make shadow pictures, bubble tube, fibre optics, kaleidoscopes.
puzzle	**Puzzles** Use a range of puzzles.
drawing	**Drawing and tracing** Drawing, colouring, stencils, tracing.
marble run	**Marble run** Watch as object moves along the marble run track.
book	**Books** Pop up books, flap books, books with lift out parts.
puppet	**Puppets** Play with hand and finger puppets.
explore	**Explore** Make binoculars using cardboard tubes. Look through cardboard tubes to focus on objects.
sort	**Sorting** Sort different shapes, colours and objects.
match	**Matching** Match objects and pictures.

Auditory exploration

Here are some possible observed behaviours that suggest the child would benefit from the following activities and from similar auditory exploratory activities. The child may find the activities motivating, and they can calm the child.

- Likes sounds to be repeated – bangs doors or objects continually, turns the TV on and off, replays TV clips
- Puts ear close to a sound to listen
- Enjoys loud noises
- Fascinated with certain sounds

hearing	SUGGESTED AUDITORY ACTIVITIES
sensory hearing	**Sensory hearing** **Make sounds with own voice** Make different sounds using the voice – humming, whispering, singing. Encourage child to be quiet and listen to silence. **Toys with sounds** Explore noisy and quiet toys.
tapping rhythms	**Tapping rhythms** Make tapping tunes. Clap, tap pencil, drum to rhythm of song.
listen and guess game	**Listen and guess game** Make sound boxes. Hide objects in containers. Suggested contents – marbles, sand, rice, shells, pasta. Shake container and guess what is inside.
musical hoops game	**Musical hoops game** Play musical hoops. Dance to music. Jump in hoop when music stops – do not make the game competitive.
sound game	**Sound game** Make animal sounds. Use 'Old Macdonald' book/song. Make animal noises for the child to guess. Listen to recordings of sounds. Play sound lotto – match picture to sound.
listening to music	**Listening to music** Listen to a range of different music. Observe the child to identify whether they find the music calming or arousing.
moving to music	**Moving to music** Move to a range of music – use streamers/scarves to encourage whole body movements. Do exercises to music.

	SUGGESTED AUDITORY ACTIVITIES
hearing	
listen to story	**Listen to story** Listen to recorded stories. Start with a story linked to the child's special interests.
sound walk	**Sound walk** Go on a sound walk. Go on outings to different environments to listen to sounds.
'wait' game	**'Wait' game** Play the 'wait' game – play music, and encourage the child to stand still when the music stops.
Simon says	**Simon says** Play 'Simon says'. Follow the verbal instructions.
guess the instrument	**Guess the instrument** Let the child explore musical instruments. Play guess the instrument – hide the instrument behind a screen and play it. See if child can recognise the instrument.
listen	**Play instruments/listen to music** Listen to music – introduce concepts of loud/quiet, start/stop, slow/fast, on/off. Allow child to turn volume of the music up and down – within safe limits.
record sounds	**Recording** Child to record sounds on the phone and listen to their recording.
compose on computer	**Computer music** Compose tunes on the computer.
rhymes and songs	**Rhymes and songs** Accompany activities with rhymes and songs throughout the day.
headphones	**Headphones** Headphones could also be used to reduce the volume of sound if the child shows sensitivity to particular sounds. Try a range of ear pieces, head phones and ear defenders.
quiet place	**Quiet place** Find a room or area in the environment that is quiet and calming for the child.

Taste exploration

Here are some possible observed behaviours that suggest the child would benefit from the following activities and from similar tasting exploratory activities. The child may find the activities motivating and they can calm the child.

- Craves certain foods
- Licks objects/people
- Likes chewing on things for long time, chews clothes, objects
- Bites others
- Chews non-edible objects
- Fascinated with certain foods

tasting	SUGGESTED TASTE EXPERIENCES
sensory taste	**Sensory taste** Provide opportunities to experience a range of foods to give different sensory experiences in the mouth. Present food in different ways. Use food in activities that do not involve eating it; e.g. use green jelly as grass for plastic animals to play in. Eat in different places. Try activities with eyes closed. Encourage the child to participate in cooking activities, snack time, food tasting, parties, festivals, picnics.
Explore different types of food	
sensory taste	**Cold foods – alerting** Ice cream, ice pops, cold drinks, frozen grapes, ice cubes.
	Crunchy textures – alerting Bread sticks, tortillas, prawn crackers, cereals, popcorn, raw vegetables, fruit such as apples.
	Chewy textures – calming Dried fruit, cereal bars, chewy sweets, cheese strings.
	Soft textures Jelly, blancmange, yoghurt, milk shakes, apple sauce, dips, custard, mashed potatoes, scrambled eggs, sandwiches, bread, pasta, noodles, rice pudding.
	Strong tasting food Give strong tasting food before getting the child to try a new food.

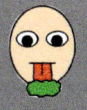 tasting	SUGGESTED TASTE EXPERIENCES
Activities involving the mouth	
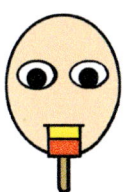 suck	**Sucking** These activities can be calming. Use a straw to drink. Drink from a sports bottle. Use a straw to suck thicker liquids such as yoghurt, fruit smoothies, purees. Suck ice cubes, ice pops, frozen fruit.
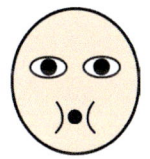 blow	**Blowing** These activities can be calming. Blow bubbles, musical instruments, whistles. Play 'blow football' with a table tennis ball, feathers, cotton wall ball or cut out paper shapes.
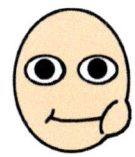 chew	**Chewing** Eating chewy foods can be calming. You can buy 'chewy tubes' which are designed to provide a resilient, non-food, chewable surface. They can provide extra sensory input and be a safe alternative for the child who craves to chew everything around them. They are made with a variety of textures and different shapes such as a chewable T shape, sticks and bracelets.
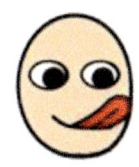 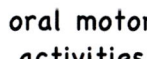 oral motor activities	**Oral motor activities** These activities encourage awareness and can alert the child. Encourage the child to copy you making different movements with your tongue. Play making funny faces in a mirror.

Smell exploration

Here are some possible observed behaviours that suggest the child would benefit from the following activities and from similar smelly exploratory activities. The child may find the activities motivating and they can calm the child.

- Need to smell themselves, others and objects
- Seeks strong odours
- Fascinated by certain smells

smelling	**SUGGESTED SMELL ACTIVITIES** **Find out personal preferences and discover which smells are calming (possibly vanilla) and which are alerting (possibly lemon).**
sensory smell	**Sensory smell** Explore foods with different smells – tea, coffee, chocolate, lemon, orange, banana, hot bread, fish. Some scents can be very calming. Put a couple of drops of essential oil or perfume on a piece of material that the child can carry with them or on a wrist band so that they can smell it if they are anxious. Make a scented pillow.
cooking	**Cooking** Participating in a cookery activity often encourages a child to smell and then try a new food.
nature walk	**Nature walk** Go on a 'smelly' walk. Go on a nature walk, town walk or seaside visit. Visit gardens and garden centres. Plant an area in the garden that has herbs and scented plants.
smelling game	**Smelling game**. Put items in containers – cover the container and ask the child to guess the smell. Suggested items – aromatherapy oils and potpourri, toiletries such as soap, shampoo, shaving foam or talc, herbs and spices.

Body awareness

Here are some possible observed behaviours that suggest the child would benefit from the following activities and from similar movement exploratory activities. The child may find the activities motivating and they can calm the child.

- Seeks fast-moving activities
- Seeks rough and tumble play
- Likes to get into small, tight places
- Likes to lean on furniture/against walls
- Fascinated by movement
- Spends a lot of time jumping
- Unable to sit still, constantly moving
- Likes to turn upside down
- Craves rocking or spinning sensations
- Paces up and down
- Always running rather than walking

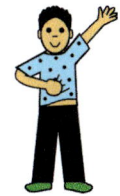	**Suggested activities for proprioceptive input**
Before a sitting activity, try some of these sensory activities. **For calming, use rhythmic movements or erratic movements to alert the child.** **It is important to note which activities calm and which alert the individual, as it easy to overarouse a child.**	
Heavy muscle activities – they help regulate input to muscles and joints and help to calm.	
Whole body	
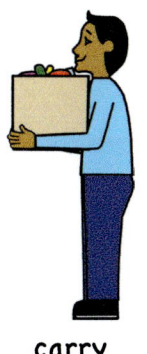 **carry**	**Carrying activities** Move or stack chairs. Wear a weighted backpack. Put weighted blanket or toy on child's knees or around shoulders. Note: consider the appropriate weight for the individual –too much weight could damage joints, etc.

pushing and pulling	**Pushing and pulling activities** Push with hands against the wall. Press hands together. Push ups. Tug of war. Move P.E. mats. Mop, sweep floor. Push wheelbarrow. Ride bike, tricycle or scooter.
jump	**Bouncing and jumping** Bounce on trampoline or mini trampoline. Bounce on large ball, space hopper. Skipping.
climb	**Climbing** Climb ladders, stairs, monkey bars, climbing frame.
Run, hop, balance	**Run, hop, balance** Create an obstacle course and encourage the child to move in different ways through it – run/jog/jump/march/hop.
exercise	**Yoga exercises** Teach the child how to stretch and relax muscles.
parachute games	**Parachute games** Parachute games are a good way to encourage movement during a fun activity.
ball	**Ball games** Practice throwing, catching and kicking a ball. Play ball games using different types and sizes of balls.

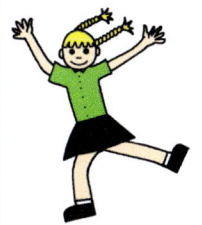	**Suggested activities for vestibular input**

Vestibular input – movement that stimulates the receptors in the inner ear.
Be careful of sensory overload.

 swing **roundabout**	**Spinning, swinging, rolling, going upside down** Swings, spinning around, roundabouts, rolling over, roll down bank.
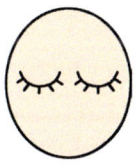 **close eyes**	**Activities with eyes closed**

The vestibular sense receives more stimulation if activities are done with eyes
closed – cover eyes and play feely box games.
Oral actions

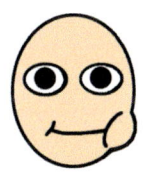 **chew**	**Chewing** Chewy tubes, chewy bracelet, chewy foods, e.g. raisins.
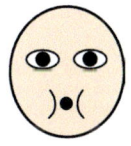 **blow**	**Blowing activities** Blow feathers. Blow bubbles. Blow paint with a straw. Play with whistles.
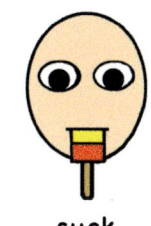 **suck**	**Sucking activities** Suck a drink through a straw. Use a sports bottle or a cup with a spout.

Using hands	
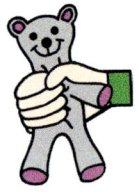 **squeeze**	**Squeezing activities** Squeeze and hug a soft toy. Squeeze play dough, clay, theraputty (firmer than play dough).
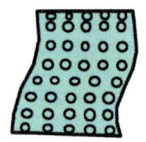 **bubble wrap**	**Bubble wrap** Use a pinching action to pop bubble wrap. Encourage play with toys and objects that require the child to make precise hand movements to develop their fine motor skills such as threading beads and building with Lego.

Relaxation	
Children with sensory processing difficulties are often anxious, find it difficult to relax and have disturbed sleep patterns, so it is important to teach relaxation strategies. Find strategies that help the child – music, soft toy cushions, bubbles, play dough, drawing or colouring, or something to squeeze such as a stress ball. Create a sensory box of items that you know calms the child.	
 relaxation CDs	**Relaxation music** Play music that child finds calming.
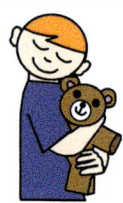 **hug**	**Hug or squeeze** Squeeze or hug toy or stress ball.
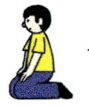 **relax**	**Relaxation sequence** Teach a sequence of relaxation activities.
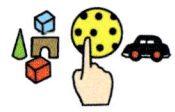 **choose**	**Choose a calming sensory activity** Choose an activity from a sensory system that the child likes and finds calming.

Reference

Department of Education (2017), *Early Years Foundation Stage Statutory Framework*, London: DfES.

7 | Resources

- Resource 7.1: letter explaining how to complete the questionnaire
- Resource 7.2: sensory observation form
- Resource 7.3: child's strengths and interests
- Resource 7.4: sensory preferences and dislikes
- Resource 7.5: grids of visual symbols
- Resource 7.6: fun activities choice board
- Resource 7.7: calming activities choice board
- Resource 7.8: an example of a completed calming activities choice board
- Resource 7.9: words for emotions
- Resource 7.10: recognising how my body feels
- Resource 7.11: Sensory Questionnaire
- Resource 7.12: visual representations

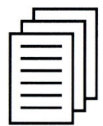

7.1 Letter explaining how to complete the questionnaire

Dear

We have attached a Sensory Questionnaire for you to complete about your child. This will help us to identify concerns and help us plan adaptations to the environment and strategies to support your child. Please complete and return to school.

Scoring

The questionnaire asks you to rank the severity of the behaviour described, with **0** being not seen and **10** being the most severe. Please use either a different colour or cross to indicate the score.

0 1 2 3 4 5 6 ⬤ 8 9 10

0 1 2 3 4 5 6 ✗ 8 9 10

Score 0 if the behaviour described is not seen.

Score between 1–4 if the behaviour described is rarely seen and is having little impact on your child's learning or daily life.

Score 5 if the behaviour is seen about once a month or is a possible barrier to learning.

Score between 6–9 if the behaviour described occurs more frequently and is a barrier to learning or significantly affects daily living.

Score 10 if the behaviour is seen throughout the day.

Please tick the right-hand box if a behaviour that is currently not causing concern was a problem in the past.

We have also included a sheet for you to indicate your child's strengths and interests, as we can use this information to plan motivators and calming activities.

If you have any questions concerning the questionnaire, please contact me at
_____.

Thank you for your help.

Yours faithfully,

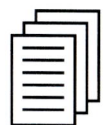

7.2 Sensory observation form

Recording your observations of the child will help you to identify the child's sensory preferences and dislikes.

Participation		Attitude		Comment
Refused to participate		Physical protest		
Resistant		Verbal protest		
Hesitant		No response		
Limited participation		Smiled		
Active participation		Laughed		
Reaction after pause in activity		**Method of communication**		
Rejected continuation of activity		Touch		
Requested different activity		Symbol		
Requested continuation of activity		Signing		
		Eye contact		
		Verbal		
Level of prompt		**Length of focus**		
Hand over hand				
Modelling				
Verbal support				
Independent				

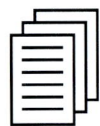

7.3 Child's strengths and interests

Things I like to touch:

Things I like to look at:

Sounds/music I like:

Things I like to eat:

Things I like to smell:

Physical activities that I like:

7.4 Sensory preferences and dislikes

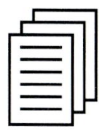

Sensory preference						
Touch	Sight	Hearing	Taste	Smell	Movement	

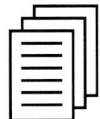

Sensory dislikes																		
Touch	**Sight**	**Hearing**	**Taste**	**Smell**	**Movement**													

7.5 Grids of visual symbols

Touch grid

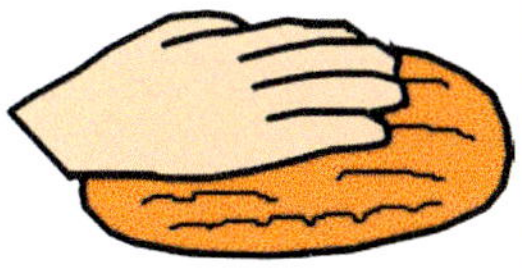 touch	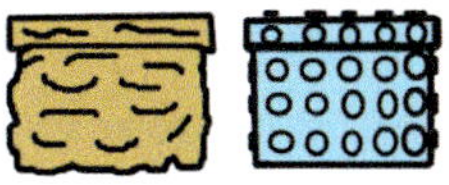 texture boxes	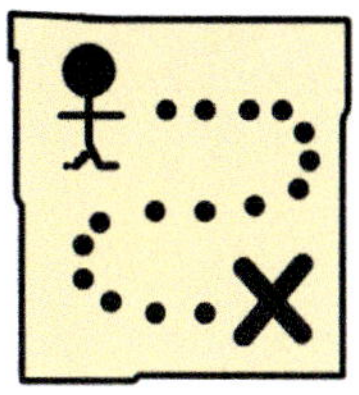 treasure hunt	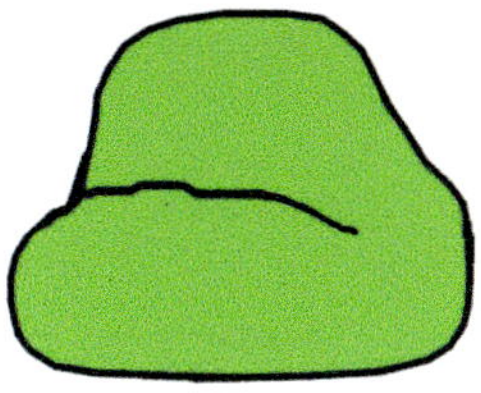 play dough
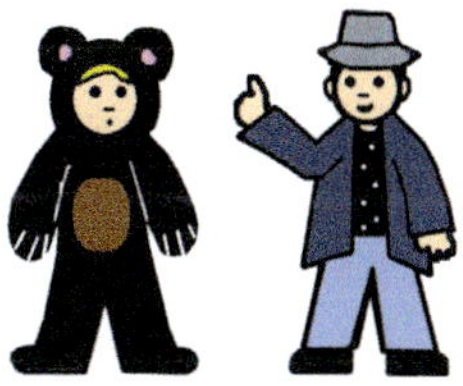 dressing up	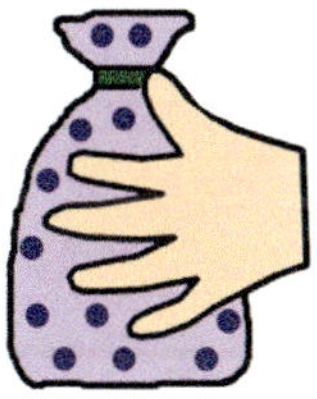 feely bag	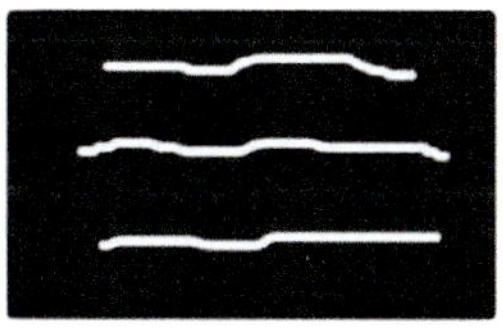 texture block game	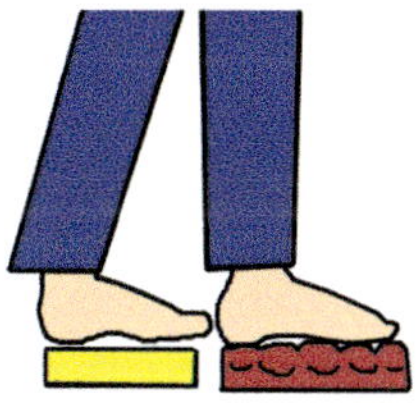 feely walk
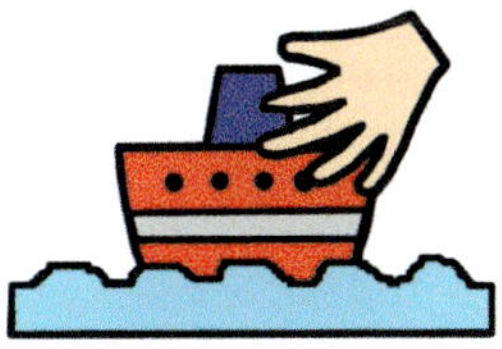 water play	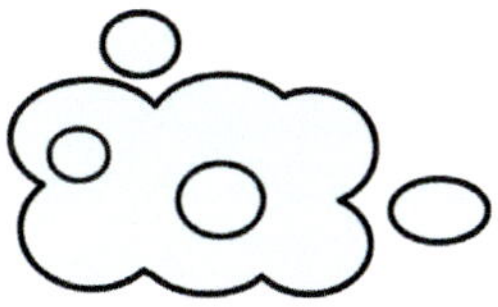 foam soap	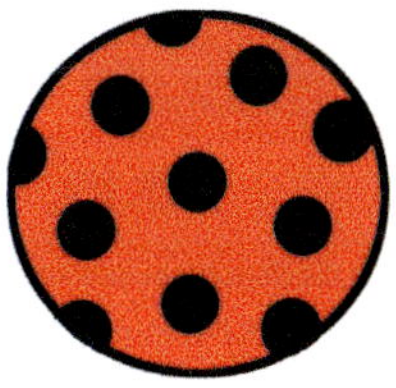 ball	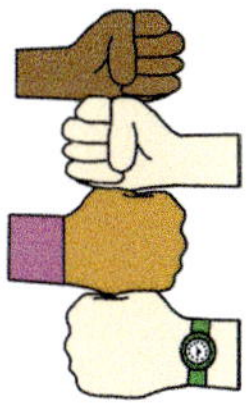 hand tower game
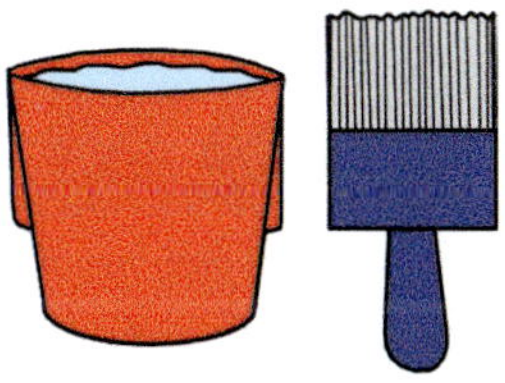 water painting	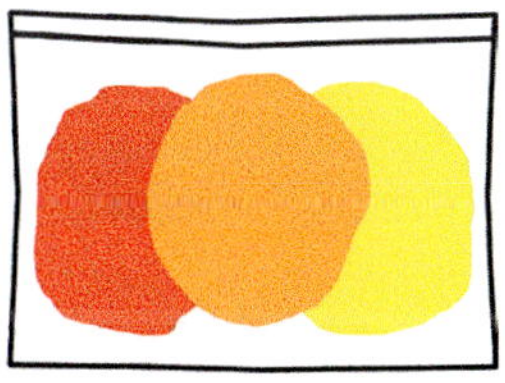 mixing colours	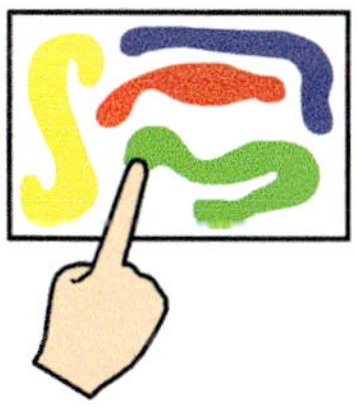 finger painting	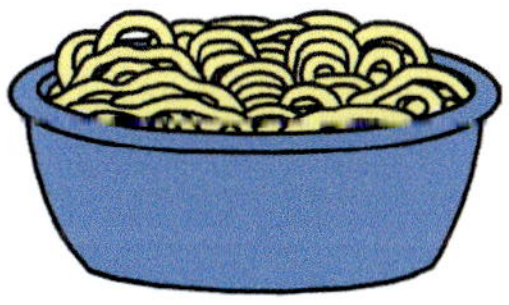 squidgy spaghetti
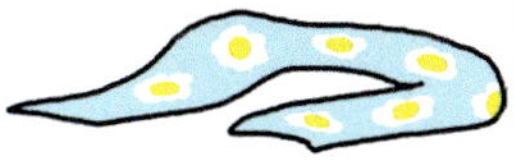 light materials	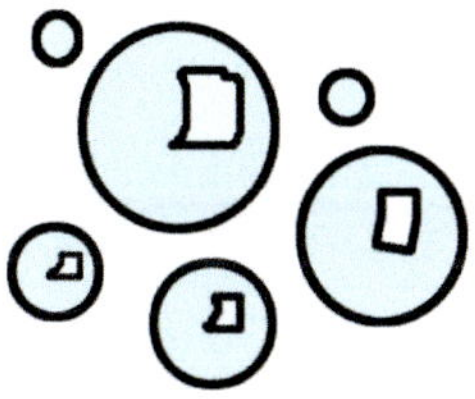 bubbles	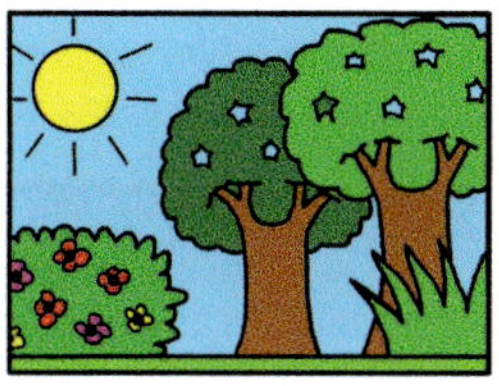 explore outside	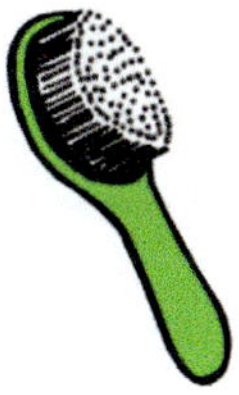 brush

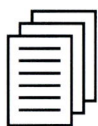

Sight grid

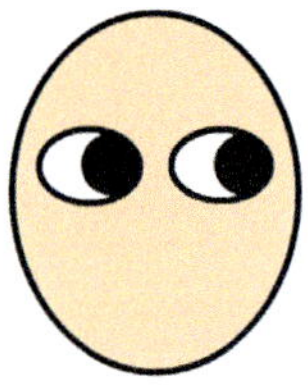 looking	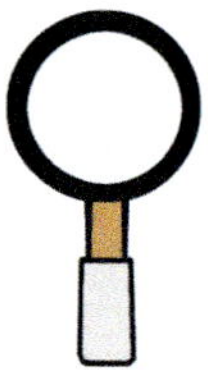 magnifying glass	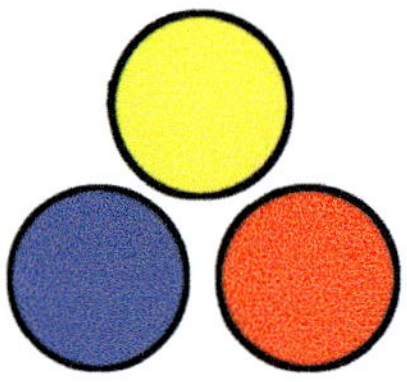 coloured looker	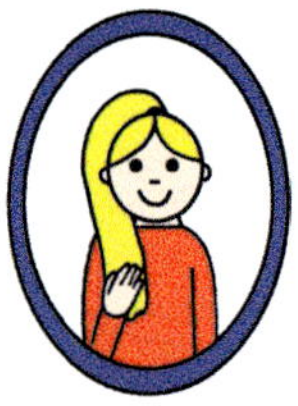 mirror
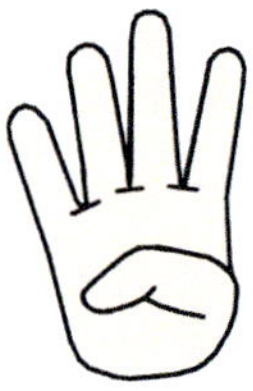 finger rhymes	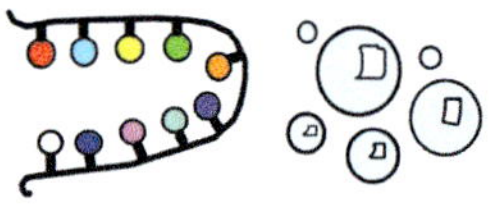 moving objects	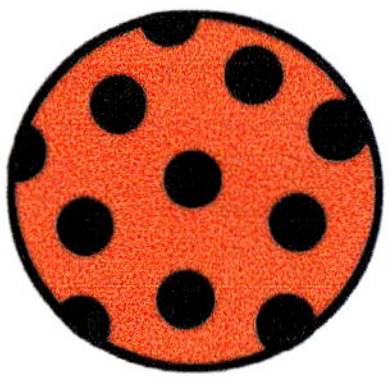 ball games	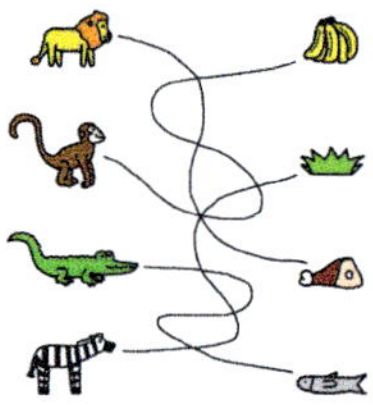 tracking
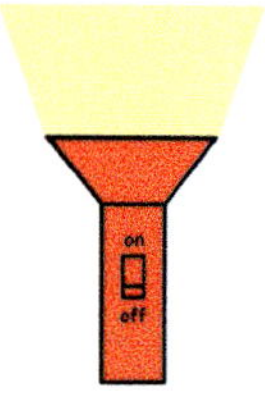 light and dark	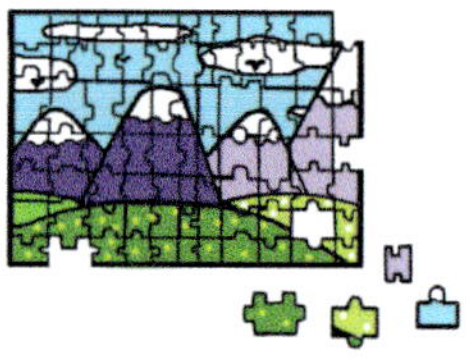 puzzle	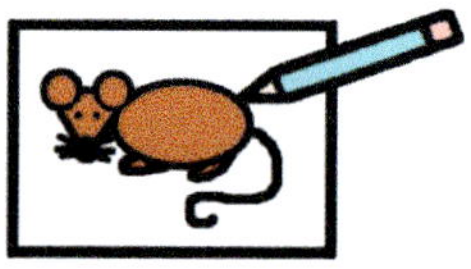 drawing	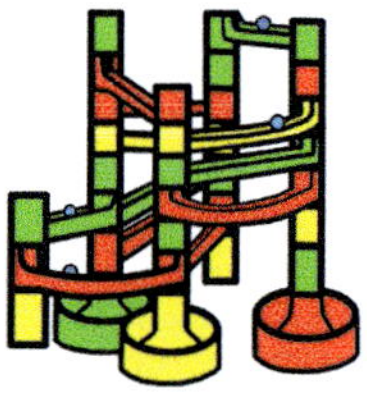 marble run
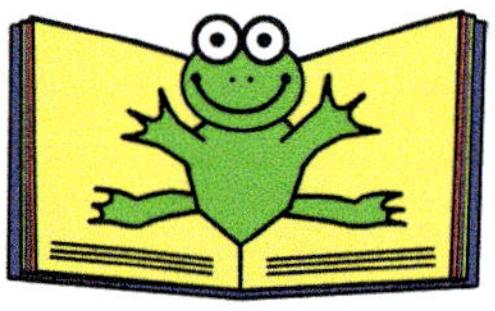 book	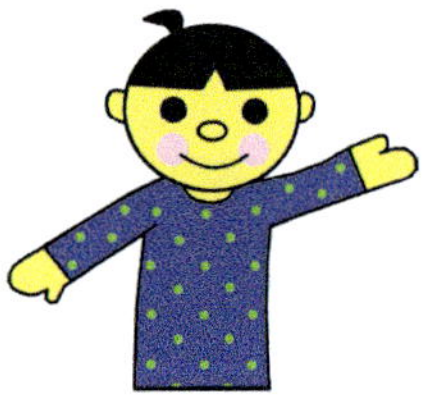 puppet	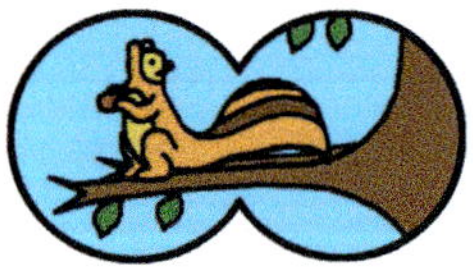 explore	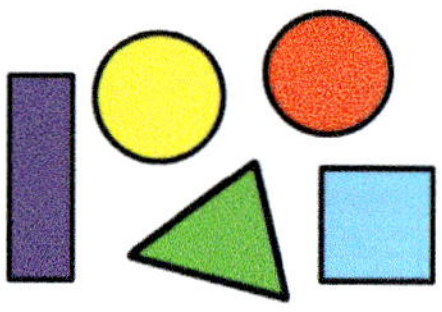 sort
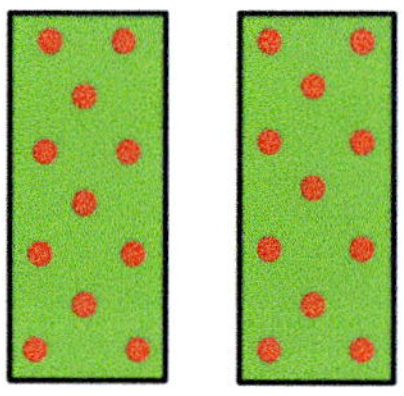 match			

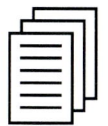

Hearing grid

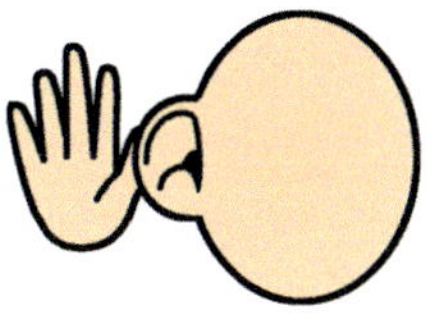 hearing	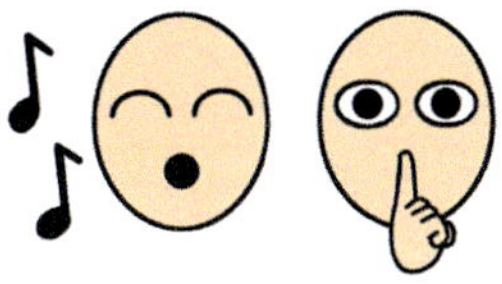 sensory hearing	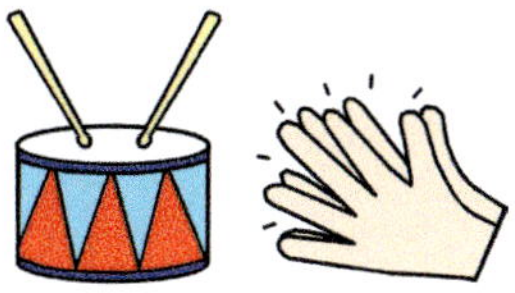 tapping rhythms	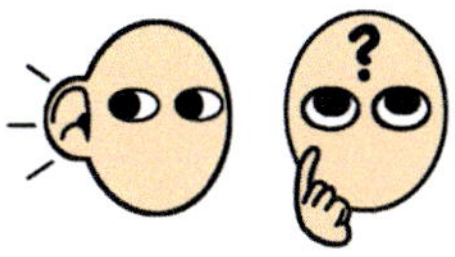 listen and guess game
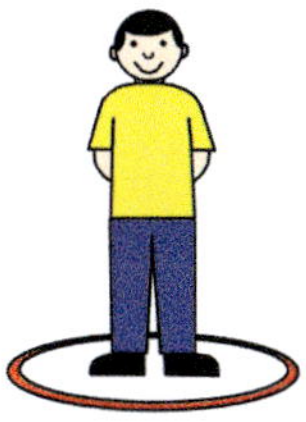 musical hoops game	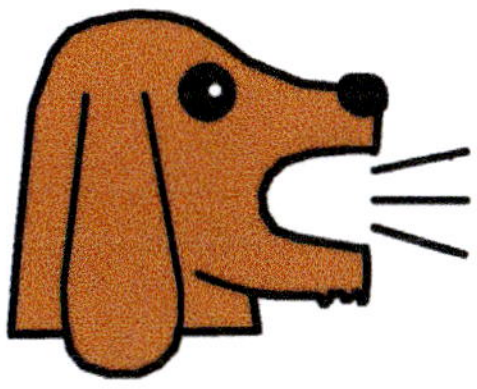 sound game	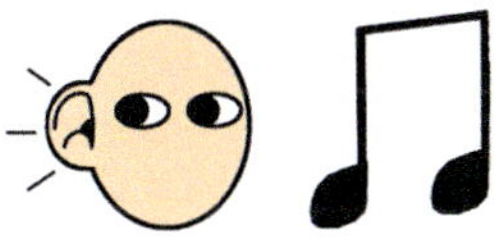 listen to music	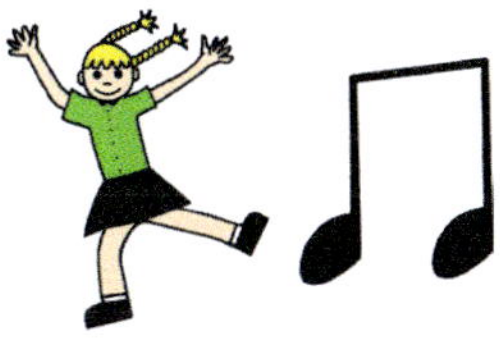 move to the music
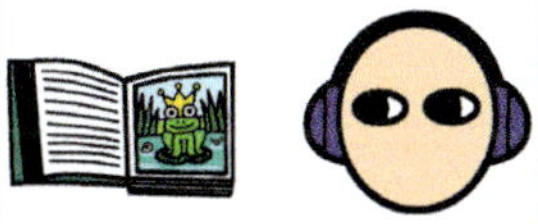 listen to story	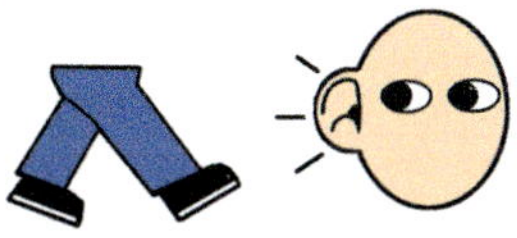 sound walk	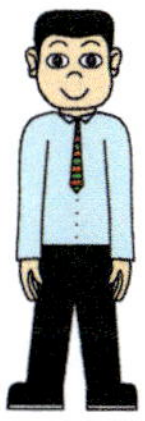 wait game	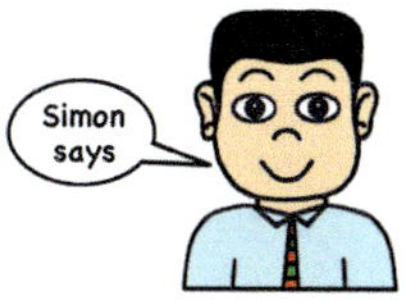 Simon says
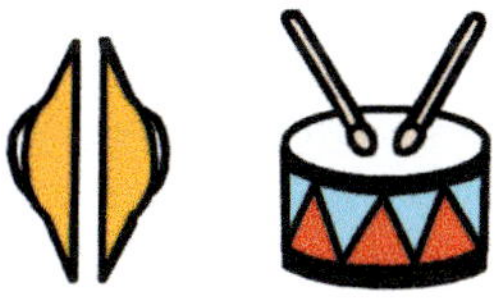 guess the instrument	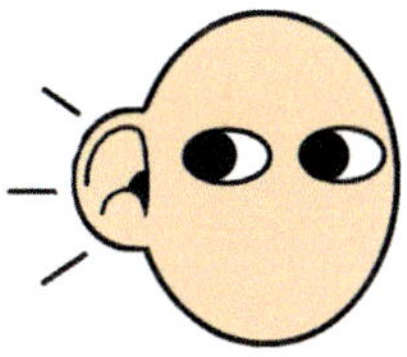 listen	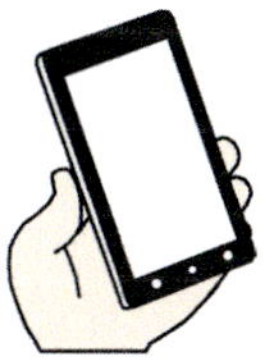 record sounds	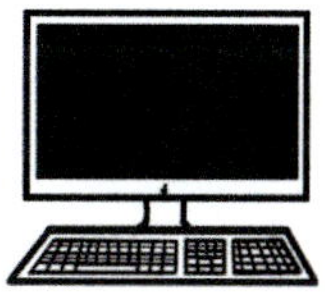 compose on computer
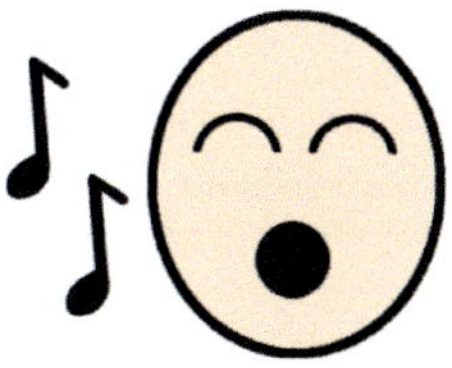 rhymes and songs	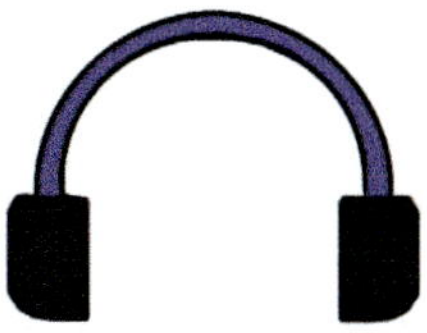 headphones	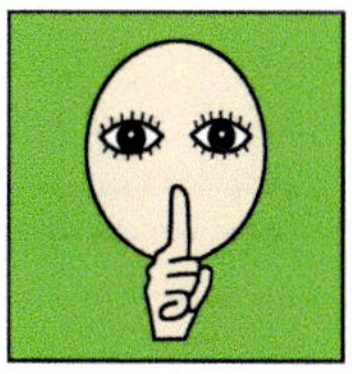 quiet place	

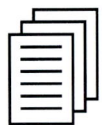

Taste grid

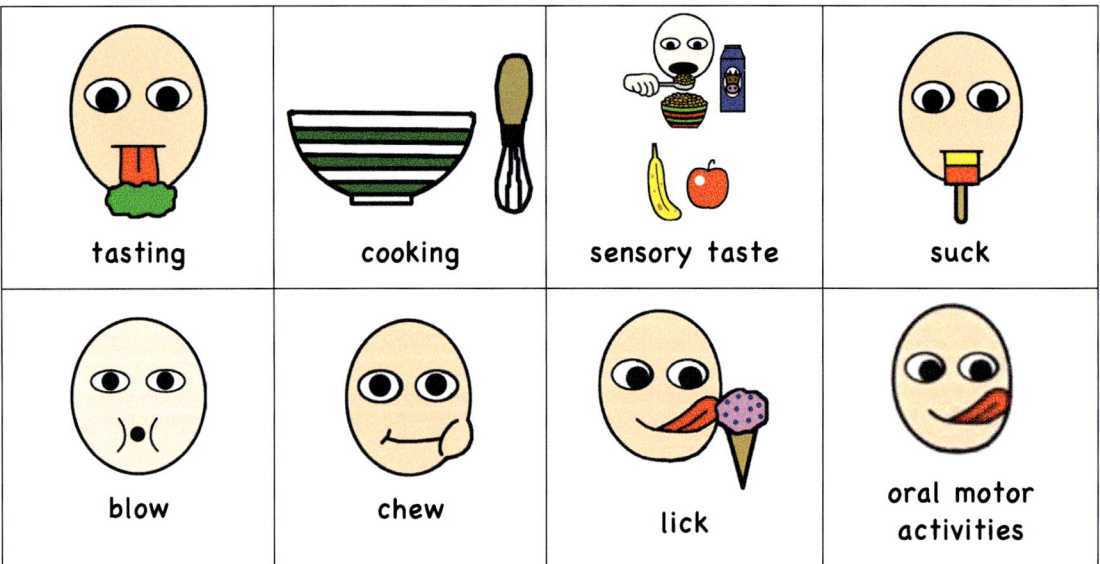

Smell grid

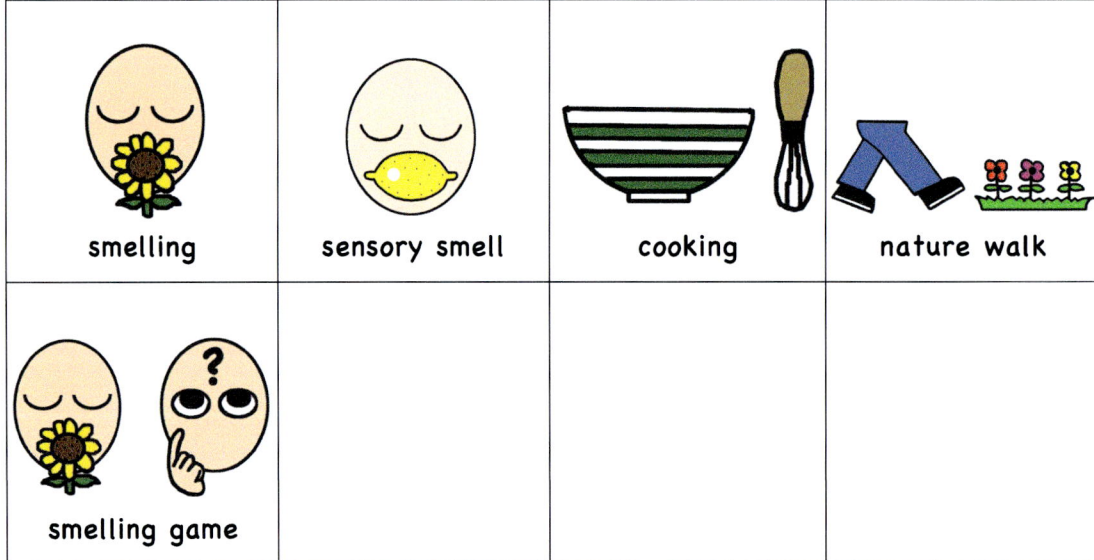

Body awareness grids

Proprioception

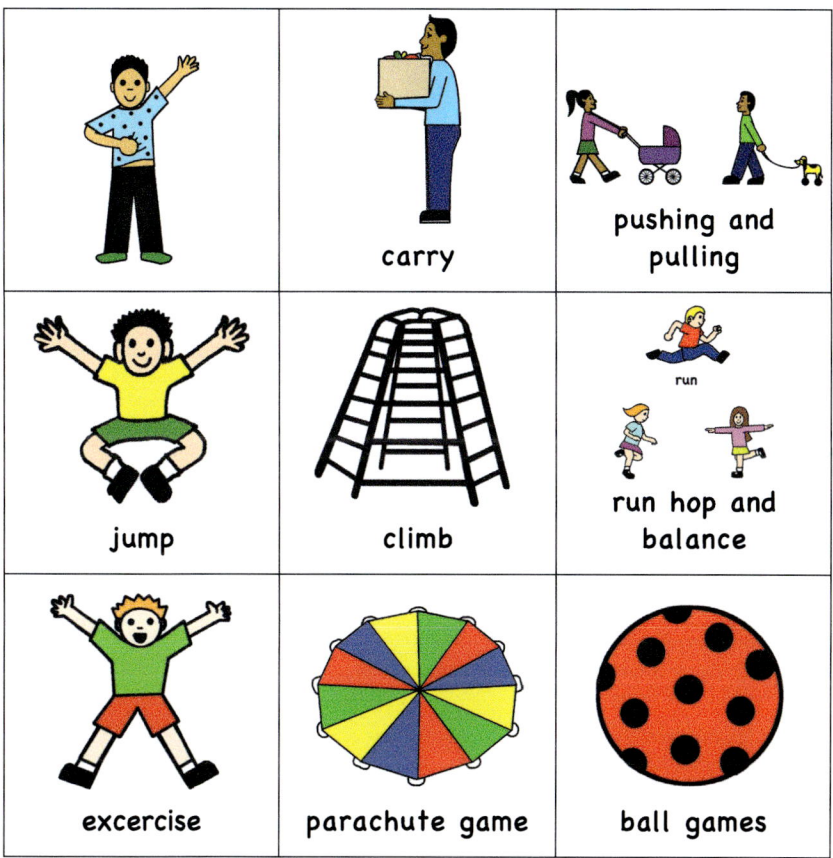

Vestibular

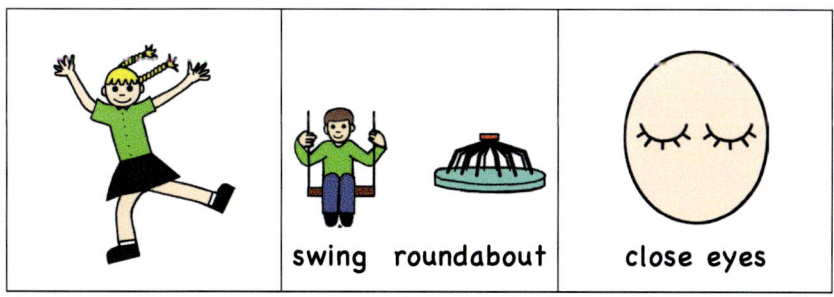

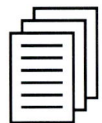

Oral actions

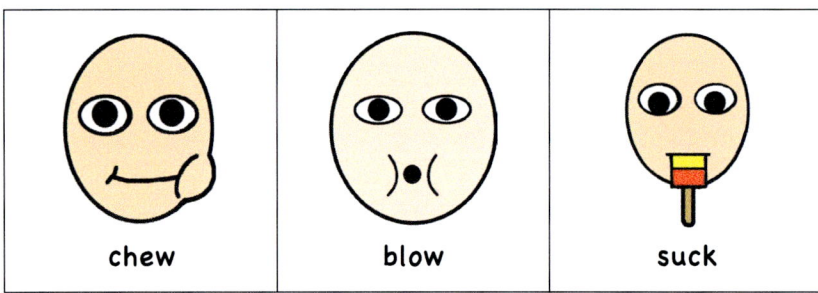

chew   blow   suck

Using hands

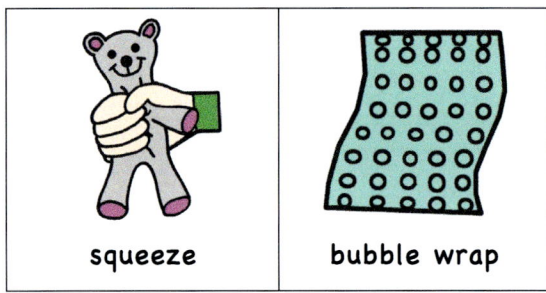

squeeze   bubble wrap

Relax

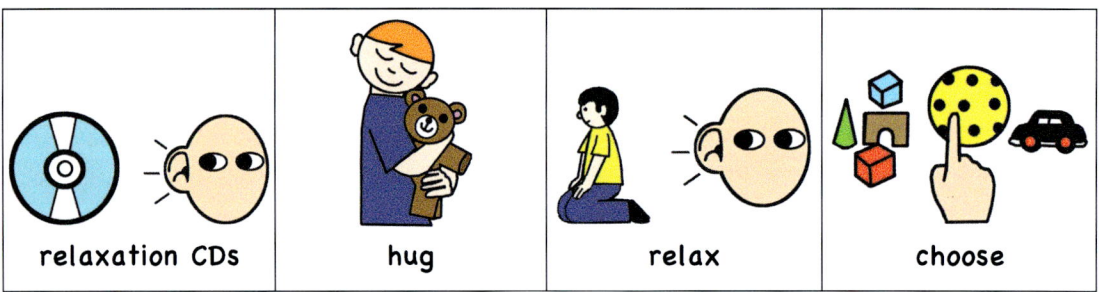

relaxation CDs   hug   relax   choose

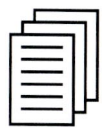

7.6 Fun activities choice board

Fun activities choice board		

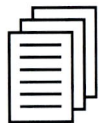

7.7 Calming activities choice board

Calming activities choice board		

7.8 An example of a completed calming activities choice board

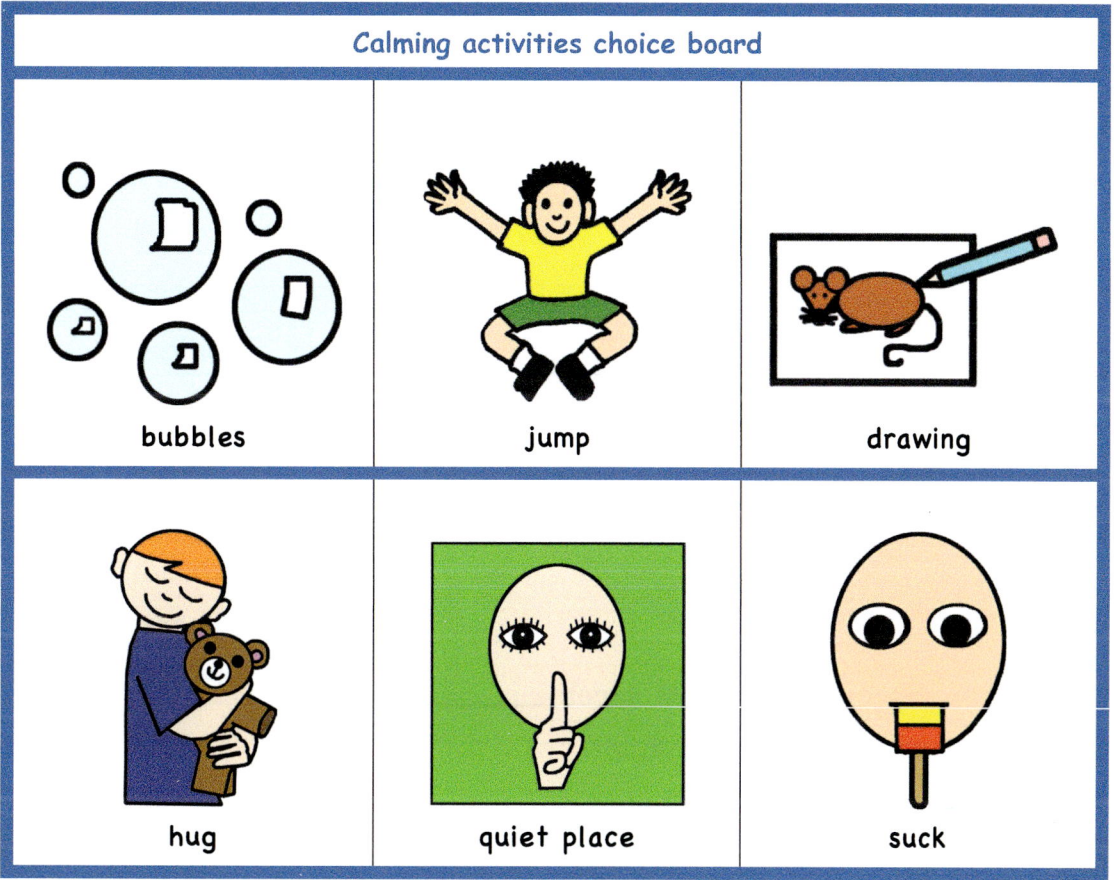

Calming activities choice board

bubbles	jump	drawing
hug	quiet place	suck

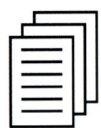

7.9 Words for emotions

How do you feel?

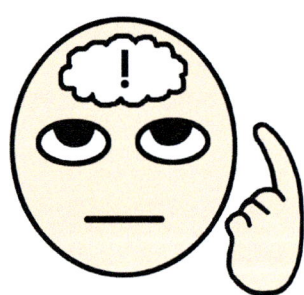

Joyful
Ecstatic
Pleased
Delighted
Cheerful
Optimistic
Happy

Thrilled
Eager
Exhilarated
Agitated
Enthusiastic
Animated
Excited

Miserable
Upset
Bored
Lonely
Depressed
Disappointed
Sad

Nervous
Agitated
Afraid
Panicky
Scared
Anxious
Worried

Fuming
Mad
Cross
Irritated
Furious
Frustrated
Angry

7.10 Some examples to help you recognise how your body feels

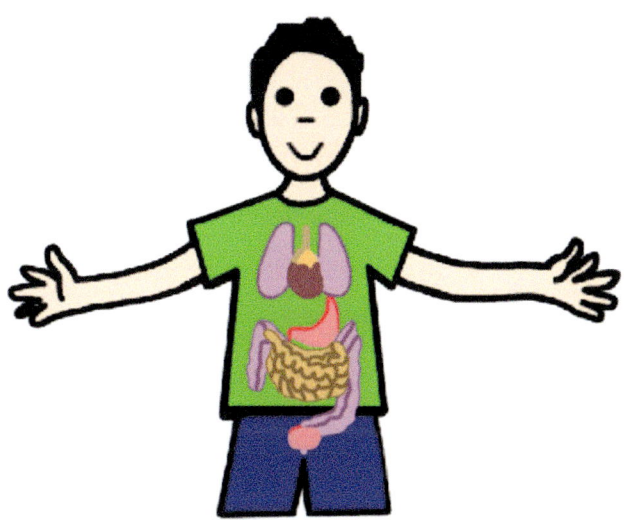

How my body feels

Think about what your body is doing	Think about why	Think about what you could do to make yourself feel more comfortable
I am sweating.	I might be ill.	I could tell an adult I do not feel well and ask them to take my temperature.
	The sun might be making me hot.	I could move out of the sun into the shade.
	I am wearing too many clothes.	I could take off my coat.

I am shivering.	I might be ill.	I could tell an adult I do not feel well and ask them to take my temperature.
	I might be cold as I am not wearing enough clothes.	I could put on my coat, scarf and gloves.

My mouth feels dry.	I might be thirsty and dehydrated.	I could get a drink.

My tummy is rumbling.	I might be hungry.	I could eat some food.

My skin feels itchy and it is red.	I may have a rash caused by an allergy to a food.	I could tell an adult and ask for some ointment.
	I may have been bitten by an insect.	I could tell an adult and ask for some ointment.
	The texture of my clothes might have been irritating my skin.	I could change my clothes.

My heart is beating fast. My legs feel wobbly. I am sweating.	I might be anxious.	I could breathe slowly and do my relaxation exercises. I could go for a walk.
	I might be ill.	I could tell an adult how I feel and ask for some medicine.

My muscles feel tight. My breathing and heart rate has increased. My face is red. I am clenching my hand.	I might be angry.	I could go to my quiet, safe place. I could suck a drink through a straw. I could wear my backpack with some heavy books in it. I could jump on my trampoline.

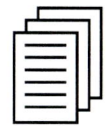

7.10 Recognising how my body feels

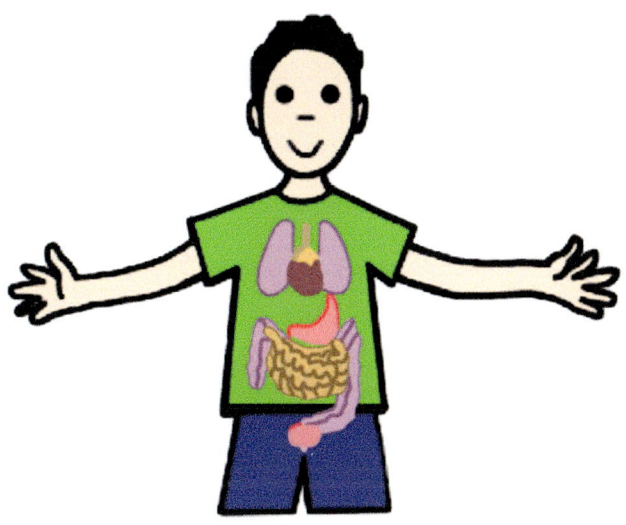

Think about what your body is doing	Think about why	Think about what you could do to make yourself feel more comfortable

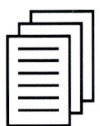

7.11 Sensory Questionnaire

CHILD'S NAME: **DATE:**

Please rate by marking **0–10** the frequency the behaviour is seen
0 = behaviour not seen, **5** = seen once a month, **10** = seen throughout the day
In the right-hand box, tick if the behaviour was a problem in the past.

TOUCH	🙂 😟
Hyperreactivity	
Light touch is painful, violently reacts to gentle touch	0 1 2 3 4 5 6 7 8 9 10 ☐
Dislikes anything on hands and feet	0 1 2 3 4 5 6 7 8 9 10 ☐
Does not like touching a range of textures	0 1 2 3 4 5 6 7 8 9 10 ☐
Avoids putting hands into messy substances	0 1 2 3 4 5 6 7 8 9 10 ☐
Does not like wearing certain textures of clothes, irritated by labels in clothes	0 1 2 3 4 5 6 7 8 9 10 ☐
Hyporeactivity	
Decreased awareness of pain – underreacts to bruises, cuts	0 1 2 3 4 5 6 7 8 9 10 ☐
Has a delayed response to textures or touch	0 1 2 3 4 5 6 7 8 9 10 ☐
Unusual interests in tactile sensory aspects of the environment	
Craves tactile stimulation	0 1 2 3 4 5 6 7 8 9 10 ☐
Self-injury – e.g. may hit head	0 1 2 3 4 5 6 7 8 9 10 ☐
Seeks very firm hugs	0 1 2 3 4 5 6 7 8 9 10 ☐
Frequently touching objects – may have routine for touching items in room	0 1 2 3 4 5 6 7 8 9 10 ☐
Fascinated by certain textures	0 1 2 3 4 5 6 7 8 9 10 ☐
Please describe the behaviour that is causing the greatest difficulty	

VISION	☺ ☹
Hyperreactivity	
Does not like particular colours	0 1 2 3 4 5 6 7 8 9 10 ☐
Avoids direct eye contact	0 1 2 3 4 5 6 7 8 9 10 ☐
Uses peripheral vision – looks at things out of the corner of the eye	0 1 2 3 4 5 6 7 8 9 10 ☐
Hits, rubs eyes when distressed	0 1 2 3 4 5 6 7 8 9 10 ☐
Overly sensitive to bright lights	0 1 2 3 4 5 6 7 8 9 10 ☐
Hyporeactivity	
Appears unaware of contrasting colours	0 1 2 3 4 5 6 7 8 9 10 ☐
Appears not to notice obstacles	0 1 2 3 4 5 6 7 8 9 10 ☐
Unusual interests in tactile sensory aspects of the environment	
Looks intently at people and objects	0 1 2 3 4 5 6 7 8 9 10 ☐
Moves head very close to objects to look at them	0 1 2 3 4 5 6 7 8 9 10 ☐
Moves fingers in front of eyes to increase stimulation	0 1 2 3 4 5 6 7 8 9 10 ☐
Fascinated with reflections	0 1 2 3 4 5 6 7 8 9 10 ☐
Fascinated with brightly coloured objects, moving patterns and colours	0 1 2 3 4 5 6 7 8 9 10 ☐
Please describe the behaviour that is causing the greatest difficulty	

AUDITORY	☺	☹
Hyperreactivity		
Able to hear sounds in the distance that others cannot hear	0 1 2 3 4 5 6 7 8 9 10 ☐	
Covers ears to block out sounds	0 1 2 3 4 5 6 7 8 9 10 ☐	
Screams in response to a particular sound	0 1 2 3 4 5 6 7 8 9 10 ☐	
Makes repetitive noises to block out sounds	0 1 2 3 4 5 6 7 8 9 10 ☐	
Dislikes noisy places	0 1 2 3 4 5 6 7 8 9 10 ☐	
Hyporeactivity		
Does not acknowledge certain sounds	0 1 2 3 4 5 6 7 8 9 10 ☐	
Has a delayed response to a sound, verbal information or instruction	0 1 2 3 4 5 6 7 8 9 10 ☐	
Unusual interests in tactile sensory aspects of the environment		
Likes sounds to be repeated – bangs doors or objects continually, turns TV on and off, replays TV clips	0 1 2 3 4 5 6 7 8 9 10 ☐	
Puts ear close to a sound to listen	0 1 2 3 4 5 6 7 8 9 10 ☐	
Enjoys loud noises	0 1 2 3 4 5 6 7 8 9 10 ☐	
Frequently makes repetitive noises; e.g. humming, clicking sounds, chants favourite words	0 1 2 3 4 5 6 7 8 9 10 ☐	
Fascinated with certain sounds	0 1 2 3 4 5 6 7 8 9 10 ☐	
Please describe the behaviour that is causing the greatest difficulty		

TASTE	☺	☹
Hyperreactivity		
Restricted diet	0 1 2 3 4 5 6 7 8 9 10 ☐	
Gags when eating certain foods	0 1 2 3 4 5 6 7 8 9 10 ☐	
Certain textures cause discomfort	0 1 2 3 4 5 6 7 8 9 10 ☐	
Does not like trying new foods, e.g. crunchy foods	0 1 2 3 4 5 6 7 8 9 10 ☐	
Shows extreme reaction when cleaning teeth	0 1 2 3 4 5 6 7 8 9 10 ☐	
Hyporeactivity		
Eats any food presented to them	0 1 2 3 4 5 6 7 8 9 10 ☐	
Shows no preference for particular tastes	0 1 2 3 4 5 6 7 8 9 10 ☐	
Unusual interests in tactile sensory aspects of the environment		
Craves certain foods	0 1 2 3 4 5 6 7 8 9 10 ☐	
Licks objects/people	0 1 2 3 4 5 6 7 8 9 10 ☐	
Likes chewing on things for a long time	0 1 2 3 4 5 6 7 8 9 10 ☐	
Chews non-edible objects	0 1 2 3 4 5 6 7 8 9 10 ☐	
Fascinated with certain foods	0 1 2 3 4 5 6 7 8 9 10 ☐	
Please describe the behaviour that is causing the greatest difficulty		

SMELL	☺	☹
Hyperreactivity		
Smells are intensified and become overpowering	0 1 2 3 4 5 6 7 8 9 10 ☐	
Strong dislike for certain smells which we may think of as pleasant	0 1 2 3 4 5 6 7 8 9 10 ☐	
Certain smells cause the child to feel nauseous	0 1 2 3 4 5 6 7 8 9 10 ☐	
Hits nose when distressed	0 1 2 3 4 5 6 7 8 9 10 ☐	
Gags when smelling certain smells	0 1 2 3 4 5 6 7 8 9 10 ☐	
Hyporeactivity		
Does not notice extreme odours	0 1 2 3 4 5 6 7 8 9 10 ☐	
Has difficulty recognising food smells	0 1 2 3 4 5 6 7 8 9 10 ☐	
Unusual interests in olfactory sensory aspects of the environment		
Needs to smell themselves and others	0 1 2 3 4 5 6 7 8 9 10 ☐	
Frequently smells objects	0 1 2 3 4 5 6 7 8 9 10 ☐	
Seeks strong odours	0 1 2 3 4 5 6 7 8 9 10 ☐	
Smells and plays with faeces	0 1 2 3 4 5 6 7 8 9 10 ☐	
Fascinated by certain smells	0 1 2 3 4 5 6 7 8 9 10 ☐	
Please describe the behaviour that is causing the greatest difficulty		

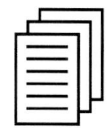

VESTIBULAR	☺	☹
Hyperreactivity		
May be frightened of activities where their feet leave the ground	0 1 2 3 4 5 6 7 8 9 10 ☐	
Avoids balancing activities	0 1 2 3 4 5 6 7 8 9 10 ☐	
Dislikes swinging activities	0 1 2 3 4 5 6 7 8 9 10 ☐	
Dislikes activities involving changes in head position	0 1 2 3 4 5 6 7 8 9 10 ☐	
Has difficulty walking on uneven surfaces	0 1 2 3 4 5 6 7 8 9 10 ☐	
Hyporeactivity		
Does not get dizzy if spins for extended amount of time	0 1 2 3 4 5 6 7 8 9 10 ☐	
Appears unaware of risks when climbing, running	0 1 2 3 4 5 6 7 8 9 10 ☐	
Unusual interests in vestibular sensory aspects of the environment		
Craves rocking or spinning sensations	0 1 2 3 4 5 6 7 8 9 10 ☐	
Frequently turns upside down	0 1 2 3 4 5 6 7 8 9 10 ☐	
Paces up and down	0 1 2 3 4 5 6 7 8 9 10 ☐	
Unable to sit still, constantly moving	0 1 2 3 4 5 6 7 8 9 10 ☐	
Craves fast movement – always running rather than walking	0 1 2 3 4 5 6 7 8 9 10 ☐	

Please describe the behaviour that is causing the greatest difficulty

PROPRIOCEPTIVE	☺	☹
Hyperreactivity		
Dislikes certain movements	0 1 2 3 4 5 6 7 8 9 10 ☐	
Difficulty with fine motor skills	0 1 2 3 4 5 6 7 8 9 10 ☐	
Dislikes fast-moving activities	0 1 2 3 4 5 6 7 8 9 10 ☐	
Child moves whole body to look at something	0 1 2 3 4 5 6 7 8 9 10 ☐	
Dislikes rough and tumble play	0 1 2 3 4 5 6 7 8 9 10 ☐	
Hyporeactivity		
Has difficulty knowing where their body is in space – unaware of position of objects and other people	0 1 2 3 4 5 6 7 8 9 10 ☐	
Unaware of how much force to use when doing a task, e.g. holds pencil too tightly	0 1 2 3 4 5 6 7 8 9 10 ☐	
Unusual interests in proprioceptive sensory aspects of the environment		
Likes to be hugged very tightly or squeezed	0 1 2 3 4 5 6 7 8 9 10 ☐	
Seeks rough and tumble play	0 1 2 3 4 5 6 7 8 9 10 ☐	
Likes to get into small, tight spaces	0 1 2 3 4 5 6 7 8 9 10 ☐	
Likes to lean on furniture/against walls	0 1 2 3 4 5 6 7 8 9 10 ☐	
Fascinated by movement	0 1 2 3 4 5 6 7 8 9 10 ☐	
Please describe the behaviour that is causing the greatest difficulty		

INTEROCEPTION	☺	☹
Hyperreactivity		
May feel pain more acutely or for longer periods of time than other people	0 1 2 3 4 5 6 7 8 9 10 ☐	
May be excessively bothered by a small injury	0 1 2 3 4 5 6 7 8 9 10 ☐	
May feel hot or cold more intensely than others	0 1 2 3 4 5 6 7 8 9 10 ☐	
Does not like the sensation of being hungry and may eat excessively to avoid the sensation	0 1 2 3 4 5 6 7 8 9 10 ☐	
Does not like the sensation of being thirsty and may drink excessively to avoid the sensation	0 1 2 3 4 5 6 7 8 9 10 ☐	
Hyporeactivity		
May not be aware of pain signals unless they are extremely intense	0 1 2 3 4 5 6 7 8 9 10 ☐	
May not recognise they are hungry or thirsty, too hot or too cold	0 1 2 3 4 5 6 7 8 9 10 ☐	
May not recognise they are ill	0 1 2 3 4 5 6 7 8 9 10 ☐	
May be aware that something is wrong but be unable to accurately identify where these sensory signals are coming from	0 1 2 3 4 5 6 7 8 9 10 ☐	
Unusual interests in interoceptive sensory aspects of the environment		
May eat excessively	0 1 2 3 4 5 6 7 8 9 10 ☐	
May drink excessively	0 1 2 3 4 5 6 7 8 9 10 ☐	
Fascinated by internal bodily sensations	0 1 2 3 4 5 6 7 8 9 10 ☐	
Please describe the behaviour that is causing the greatest difficulty		

7.12 Visual representations

TOUCH

HYPERREACTIVE

	10	9	8	7	6	5	4	3	2	1	0
Light touch is painful											
Dislikes anything on hands and feet											
Does not like touching a range of textures											
Avoids putting hands into messy substances											
Does not like wearing certain textures of clothing											

HYPOREACTIVE

	10	9	8	7	6	5	4	3	2	1	0
Decreased awareness of pain											
Delayed response to textures or touch											

SENSORY SEEKING

	10	9	8	7	6	5	4	3	2	1	0
Craves tactile stimulation											
Self-injures											
Seeks very firm hugs											
Frequently touching objects											
Fascinated by certain textures											

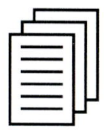

VISION

Scale: 10, 9, 8, 7, 6, 5, 4, 3, 2, 1, 0

HYPERREACTIVE
- Does not like particular colours
- Avoids direct eye contact
- Uses peripheral vision
- Hits, rubs eyes when distressed
- Overly sensitive to bright lights

HYPOREACTIVE
- Appears unaware of contrasting colours
- Appears not to notice obstacles

SENSORY SEEKING
- Looks intently at people and objects
- Moves head very close to objects to look at them
- Moves fingers in front of eyes to increase stimulation
- Fascinated with reflections
- Fascinated with brightly coloured objects, moving patterns and colours

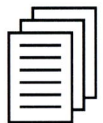

AUDITORY

HYPERREACTIVE

	Able to hear sounds in the distance others can't hear	Covers ears to block out sounds	Screams in response to particular sounds	Makes repetitive noises to block out sounds	Dislikes noisy places
10					
9					
8					
7					
6					
5					
4					
3					
2					
1					
0					

HYPOREACTIVE

	Does not acknowledge certain sounds	Has a delayed response to a sound, verbal information or instruction
10		
9		
8		
7		
6		
5		
4		
3		
2		
1		
0		

SENSORY SEEKING

	Likes sounds to be repeated	Puts ear close to a sound to listen	Enjoys loud noises	Frequently makes repetitive noises	Fascinated by certain sounds
10					
9					
8					
7					
6					
5					
4					
3					
2					
1					
0					

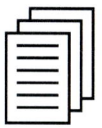

TASTE

	10	9	8	7	6	5	4	3	2	1	0
HYPERREACTIVE											
Restricted diet											
Gags when eating certain foods											
Certain textures cause discomfort											
Does not like trying new foods											
Shows extreme reaction when cleaning teeth											
HYPOREACTIVE											
Eats any food presented to them											
Shows no preference for particular tastes											
SENSORY SEEKING											
Craves certain foods											
Licks objects or people											
Likes chewing on things for a long time											
Chews non-edible objects											
Fascinated by certain foods											

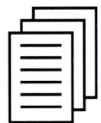

SMELL

HYPERREACTIVE

Scale	Smells are intensified and become over powering	Strong dislike for certain smells which we may think of as pleasing	Certain smells cause the child to feel nauseous	Hits nose when distressed	Gags when smelling certain smells
10					
9					
8					
7					
6					
5					
4					
3					
2					
1					
0					

HYPOREACTIVE

Scale	Does not notice extreme odours	Has difficulty recognising food smells
10		
9		
8		
7		
6		
5		
4		
3		
2		
1		
0		

SENSORY SEEKING

Scale	Needs to smell themselves and others	Frequently smells objects	Seeks strong odours	Smells and plays with faeces	Fascinated by certain smells
10					
9					
8					
7					
6					
5					
4					
3					
2					
1					
0					

VESTIBULAR

HYPERREACTIVE

	Frightened of activities where feet leave the ground	Avoids balancing activities	Dislikes swinging activities	Dislikes activities involving changes in head position	Has difficulty walking on uneven surfaces
10					
9					
8					
7					
6					
5					
4					
3					
2					
1					
0					

HYPOREACTIVE

	Doesn't get dizzy if spins for extended amount of time	Appears unaware of risks when climbing or running
10		
9		
8		
7		
6		
5		
4		
3		
2		
1		
0		

SENSORY SEEKING

	Craves rocking or spinning sensations	Frequently turns upside down	Paces up and down	Unable to sit still, constantly moving	Craves fast movement; always running rather than walking
10					
9					
8					
7					
6					
5					
4					
3					
2					
1					
0					

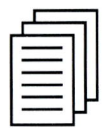

PROPRIOCEPTION

HYPERREACTIVE

	10	9	8	7	6	5	4	3	2	1	0
Dislikes certain movements											
Difficulty with fine motor activities											
Dislikes fast moving activities											
Moves whole body to look at something											
Dislikes rough and tumble play											

HYPOREACTIVE

	10	9	8	7	6	5	4	3	2	1	0
Has difficulty knowing where their body is in space											
Unaware of how much force to use when doing a task											

SENSORY SEEKING

	10	9	8	7	6	5	4	3	2	1	0
Likes to be hugged very tightly or squeezed											
Seeks rough and tumble play											
Likes to get into small, tight places											
Likes to lean on furniture or against walls											
Fascinated by movement											

INTEROCEPTION

HYPERREACTIVE

Scale	Descriptions
10, 9, 8, 7, 6, 5, 4, 3, 2, 1, 0	May feel pain more acutely or for longer periods of time
	May be overly bothered by a small injury
	May feel hot or cold more intensely than others
	Does not like the sensation of being hungry
	Does not like the sensation of being thirsty

HYPOREACTIVE

Scale	Descriptions
10, 9, 8, 7, 6, 5, 4, 3, 2, 1, 0	May not be aware of pain signals unless extremely intense
	May not recognise they are hungry or thirsty
	May not recognise they are ill
	May be aware that something is wrong but be unable to identify where sensory signals are coming from

SENSORY SEEKING

Scale	Descriptions
10, 9, 8, 7, 6, 5, 4, 3, 2, 1, 0	May eat excessively
	May drink excessively
	Fascinated by internal bodily sensations

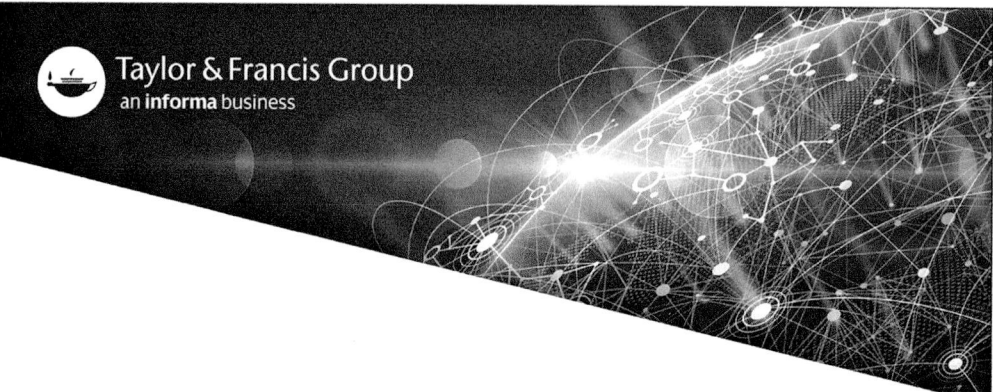
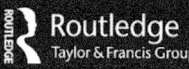
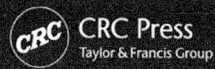